HEALTH PROMOTION & DISEASE PREVENTION

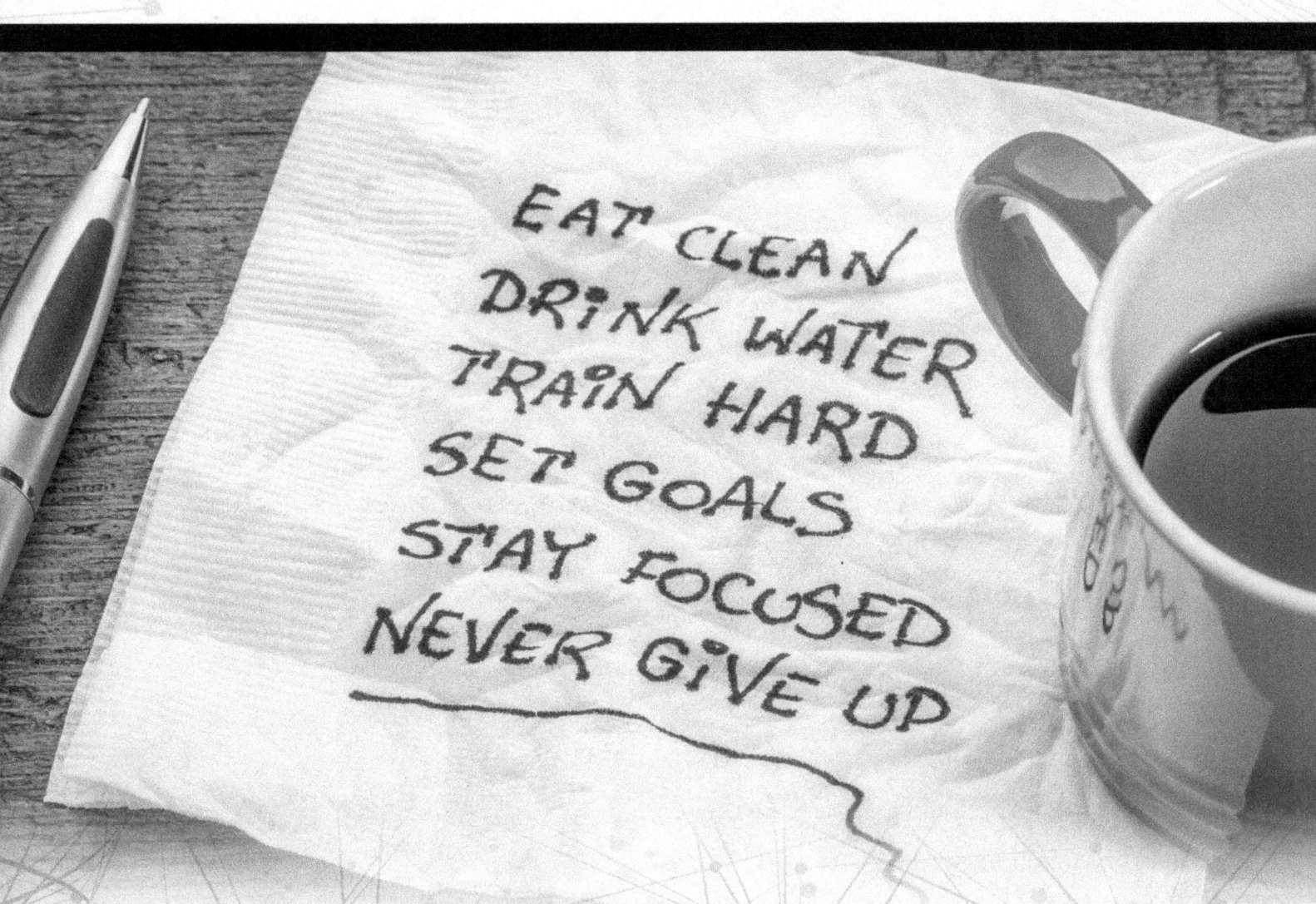

Kendall Hunt
publishing company

Dr. Lana Zinger

Queensborough Community College

Cover image © Shutterstock.com
Previously sold as *Healthy Happy Long Life*, 2nd Edition and *Building Healthy Communities*, 2nd Edition

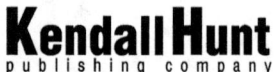

www.kendallhunt.com
Send all inquires to:
4050 Westmark Drive
Dubuque, IA 52004-1840

Copyright © 2019 by Kendall Hunt Publishing Company

ISBN 978-1-5249-7095-6

Published in the United States of America

··

Health, the greatest of all we count as blessings.
—Ariphron

··

To my sons Max and Alex who have greatly enriched my life with their healthy attitudes, spirited personalities and unconditional love. To my mom who taught me strength, perseverance, and to never give up.

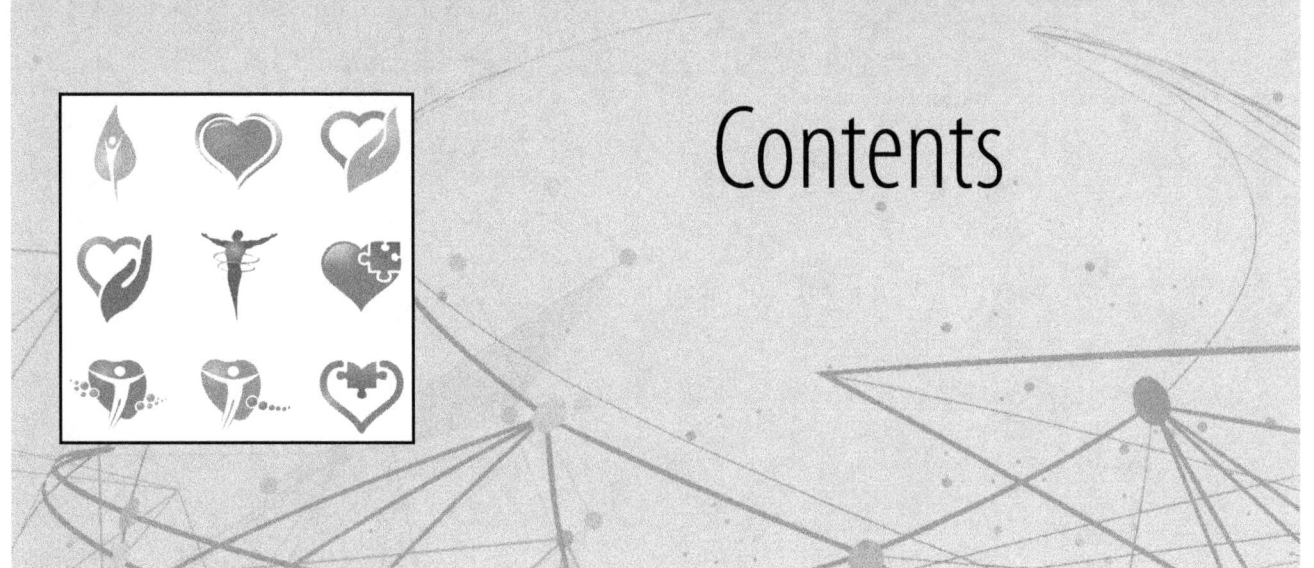

Contents

Beginning of semester questions:

Based on your own experiences, answer the questions 24 – 26 using the one of the following five choices:

(a) strongly agree
(b) agree
(c) neither agree nor disagree
(d) disagree
(e) strongly disagree

24. My awareness of health issues is important to me.

agree

25. I have the capability to make informed health decisions.

agree

26. I make healthy lifestyle choices.

agree

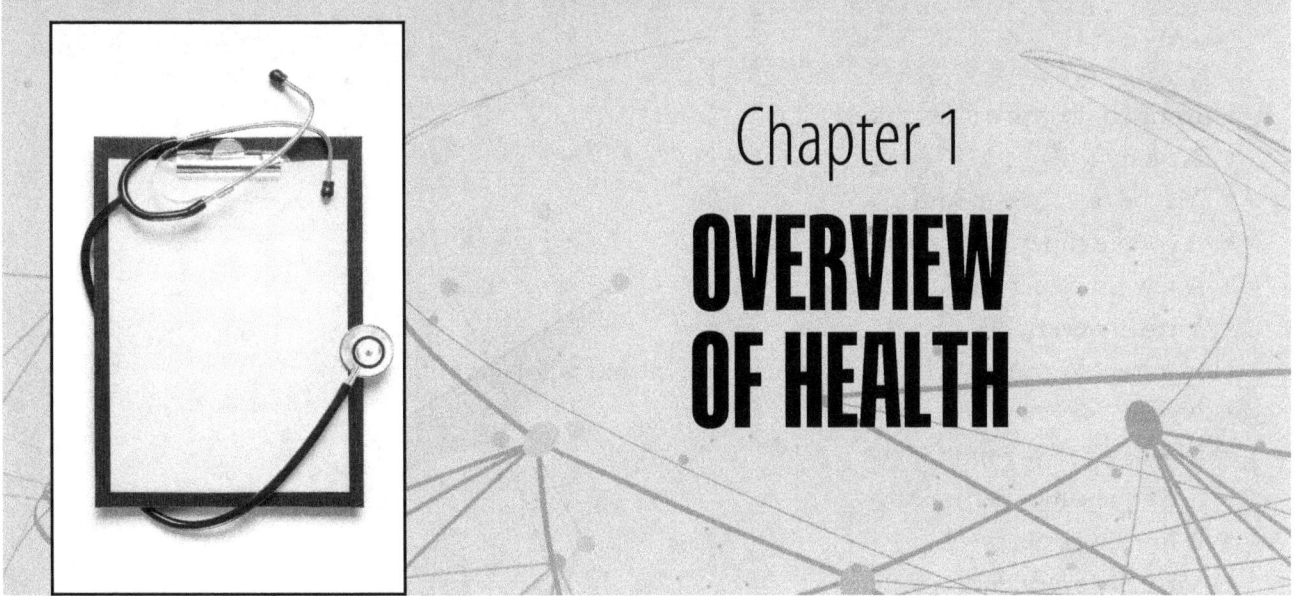

Chapter 1

OVERVIEW OF HEALTH

How Healthy Are You?

1. How much extra weight are you carrying around (be honest)?
   - None at all
   - I have a few extra pounds
   - More than 10 pounds
   - I am seriously overweight
2. How much regular exercise do you get?
   - None at all
   - A few times per week
   - Almost every day
3. How much TV/Internet time do you spend a day?
   - None
   - 1–2 hours
   - 3–5 hours
   - 6–8 hours
   - 8+ hours
4. How many meals do you eat per day?
   - 1
   - 2
   - 3
   - More than 3

5. How often do you eat fast food?
   - Never
   - Maybe once per month
   - A couple times per month
   - A few times per week
   - Virtually every day
6. How often do you eat whole grains, oats, cereal and wholegrain bread?
   - Never
   - Maybe once per month
   - A couple times per month
   - A few times per week
   - Virtually every day
7. How many servings of fruit and vegetables do you eat each a day?
   - 5+
   - 3, 4
   - 1, 2
   - Virtually never
8. Do you watch your salt intake?
   - Never
   - Yes, I read food labels
   - I don't use any added salt
9. Apart from coffee or tea, what do you usually drink during the day?
   - Water
   - Soda/diet soda
   - Fruit juice
   - Sports drinks
10. Do you take a daily vitamin?
    - Every day
    - Most days
    - Some days
    - Never
11. Are you a smoker?
    - Not at all, never was
    - No, I quit
    - I am a social smoker
    - A few cigarettes per day
    - At least one pack per day
12. Do you live or work with a smoker?
    - Yes
    - No

13. How much alcohol do you drink per week?
    - None at all
    - A few drinks per week
    - I drink heavily a few times per week
    - I have a few drinks every day
    - I drink pretty heavily every day
14. Do you use "recreational" drugs?
    - Never
    - From time to time
    - Probably once a week
    - Very regularly
15. What is your level of school stress?
    - None really
    - A little bit here and there
    - I have pretty regular stress at school
    - Almost every minute of the day at school is stressful for me
16. What is your level of home stress?
    - None really
    - A little bit here and there
    - I have pretty regular stress at home
    - Almost every minute of the day at home is stressful for me
17. What is your outlook on life?
    - I have a very happy disposition
    - I'm a cautious optimist
    - I am skeptical about a lot of stuff
    - I require a lot of evidence but then I embrace good things
    - I think the world is pretty much all crap all the time
18. Do you have any family history of heart disease?
    - Yes
    - No
19. Has anyone in your immediate family suffered a stroke before the age of 50?
    - Yes
    - No
20. Has anyone in your family been diagnosed with cancer?
    - Yes
    - No
21. Has anyone in your family been diagnosed with diabetes?
    - Yes
    - No
22. Based on the above answers, do you think you are healthy?
    - Yes
    - No

23. Why or why not?

_____

_____

_____

_____

_____

24. Which area(s) if any, do you think you should work on improving?

_____

_____

_____

_____

_____

25. Name the most important health concerns facing you, your community, family, and/or friends:

_____

_____

_____

_____

_____

Definitions of Health and Wellness

Health is a subjective concept that is defined in relationship to cultural values and social norms. The World Health Organization defines health as being sound in body, mind, and spirit. It is not merely the absence of disease or infirmity, but a state of complete physical, mental, and social well-being.[1] A Report of the Surgeon General states that health means being physically fit enough to have mental functions of thinking, reasoning, feeling, and thoughts about purposive behavior.[2] Similarly, wellness is defined as a deliberate lifestyle choice characterized by personal responsibility and optimal enhancement of physical, mental, and spiritual health.

4

Components of Health

1. Physical—nutrition (food/weight/BMI)
2. Emotional—expression and control of emotions; self-esteem
3. Environmental—appreciation of external environment and your role in improving and protecting your surroundings
4. Intellectual—ability to think, analyze, and use brain power successfully and effectively in dealing with situations
5. Spiritual—hopes for life; what your existence means
6. Social—interactions with others

Global health is concerned with health that crosses national borders. Global health is a huge concern because modern transportation allows infectious diseases to spread across the world in an alarming rate.

Public health is the sum of all governmental efforts to promote, protect, and preserve the people's health. Public health is concerned with threats to the overall health of a community based on population health analysis. The population in question can be as big as a handful of people or several continents.

• Environmental, social, behavioral, and occupational health, are also important fields in public health.

The developing world still suffers from largely preventable infectious diseases, mainly caused by malnutrition and poverty. Discrepancies regarding access to health care and public health initiatives between developed nations and developing nations still exist, and a large majority of disease and mortality in the developing world results from and contributes to extreme poverty. One of the most relevant factors for increased preventable diseases globally is that many public health infrastructures are still in the process of formation throughout the world. Another concern is that not enough trained health workers or monetary resources are available to provide medical care or to work at disease prevention.

The focus of a public health intervention is to prevent rather than treat a disease, especially through the promotion of healthy behaviors. Examples of public health measures include vaccination programs and distribution of condoms.

Life Expectancy

The average number of years a newborn is expected to live with current mortality patterns remaining the same.

United States = 78.4 years of age

As of September 23, 2010, the United States currently ranks 49th in the world in overall life expectancy, according to a study published in the Journal of Health Affairs, slipping dramatically during the last decade. The decline is highlighted by the fact that in 1999, the World Health Organization ranked the U.S. as 24th in the world in life expectancy. Obesity, smoking, traffic fatalities, and homicide are strong reasons for this low rank, but a recent study zoned in on flaws in the nation's health care system as the main culprit.

The study, "What Changes in Survival Rates Tell Us about U.S. Health Care," which was funded by the Commonwealth Fund, found that failings in the U.S. health care system, such as costly specialized and fragmented care, are likely playing a large role in this relatively poor performance on improvements in life expectancy. The United States spends over twice as much per capita on health care than other industrialized nations, so why do we have shorter life expectancies?

All the focus is on profit instead of focusing on preventive care, wellness, healthy food and water, and a safe environment.

Factors for Increased Life Expectancy

- Vaccinations
- Control of infectious diseases
- Fluoridation of drinking water
- Pasteurization of milk
- Safer storage of food
- Safer workplaces
- Motor vehicle safety

Top 10 Leading Causes of Death for All Ages in the United States[3]

1. Heart disease
2. Cancer
3. Stroke
4. Lung disease
5. Diabetes
6. Influenza/pneumonia
7. Alzheimer's disease
8. Motor vehicle (MV) crashes
9. Kidney disease
10. Septicemia (systemic blood infection)

Top 10 Leading Causes of Death for Young Adults in the United States[4]

1. MV crashes
2. Homicide
3. Suicide
4. Accidental poisoning
5. Cancer
6. Heart disease
7. Accidental drowning
8. Congenital abnormalities
9. Accidental falls
10. HIV/AIDS

The Centers for Disease Control and Prevention's (CDC) Six Critical Health Behaviors:

1. **Cigarette smoking** accounts for approximately 1 of every 5 deaths, or about 400,000 people. Each day in the United States, approximately 3,600 young people between the ages of 12 and 17 years start cigarette smoking.

2. **Unhealthy eating** is associated with increased risk for many diseases, including the three leading causes of death: heart disease, cancer, and stroke. In 2009, only 22.3 percent of high school students reported eating fruits and vegetables five or more times during the past 7 days.

3. **Inadequate physical activity** increases the risk of premature death and diseases such as heart disease, hypertension, cancer, and diabetes. Regular physical activity in childhood and adolescence improves academic performance, especially memory retention, strength and endurance, helps build healthy bones and muscles, helps control weight, reduces anxiety and stress, increases self-esteem, and improves blood pressure and cholesterol levels. The U.S. Department of Health and Human Services recommends that young people participate in at least 60 minutes of physical activity *daily*.

4. **Unsafe sexual behaviors.** Vaginal, anal, and oral intercourse place young people at risk for HIV infection and other sexually transmitted diseases (STDs).

5. **Alcohol and drug use**
   - Alcohol is **one of the most widely used drug substances** in the world. Alcohol is used by more young people in the United States than tobacco or illicit drugs. Excessive alcohol consumption is associated with approximately 75,000 deaths per year.
   - Long-term alcohol misuse is associated with liver disease, cancer, cardiovascular disease, and neurological damage as well as psychiatric problems such as depression, anxiety, and antisocial personality disorder.
   - Marijuana is the most commonly used illicit drug among youth in the United States.
   - Prescription and over-the-counter (OTC) drug abuse remain high. Prescription medications most commonly abused by youth include pain relievers, tranquilizers, stimulants, and depressants. In 2009, 20 percent of U.S. high school students reported taking a prescription drug, such as Oxycontin, Percocet, Vicodin, Adderall, Ritalin, or Xanax, without a doctor's prescription. Teens also misuse OTC cough and cold medications containing the cough suppressant dextromethorphan (DXM), such as Robitussin, to get high.

6. **Injury and violence** are the leading cause of death and disability for people aged 1 to 44 years. Approximately 72 percent of all deaths among adolescents aged 10–24 years are attributed to injuries from four causes: motor vehicle crashes (30%), all other unintentional injuries (15%), homicide (15%), and suicide (12%). Highly associated with these injuries are adolescent behaviors such as physical fights, carrying weapons, making a suicide plan, and not using seatbelts.

What is a Healthy Community?

A Healthy Community: Meets basic needs of all

- Affordable, safe, accessible, and nutritious foods
- Affordable, high quality housing
- Affordable, accessible, and high quality health care
- Affordable and high quality schools, parks and recreational facilities, child care, libraries, and playgrounds
- Access, affordable, and safe opportunities for physical activity

- Clean air, soil and water, and environment
- Green and open spaces
- Minimized toxics, emissions, and waste
- Affordable and sustainable energy use
- Living wage, safe and healthy job opportunities for all
- Opportunities for all to have a high quality and accessible education
- Socially cohesive and supportive relationships, families, homes, and neighborhoods
- Safe communities, free of crime and violence

Does this describe your community?

_____

_____

_____

_____

How can you support your community?

- Support local farmers markets and other access points to fresh fruits and vegetables.
- Inquire about volunteer opportunities at community health centers.
- Partner with local parks and recreational facilities to increase access to safe places to be outside and physically active.
- Work with local authorities to initiate violence intervention and prevention efforts.
- Volunteer to speak about the importance of public health and prevention at local schools, houses of worship, workplaces, and community organizations.
- Create a local health movement! Start a healthy food co-op, organize a canning circle, gather a walking group, or form a club dedicated to volunteering.

What is Healthy People 2020?[5]

It is the government's 10-year national objectives for improving the health of all Americans. Read www.HealthyPeople.gov.ure progress, and their importance as public health issues.

Four Goals of Healthy People 2020:

- Attain high-quality, longer lives free of preventable disease, disability, injury, and premature death;

- Achieve health equity, eliminate disparities, and improve the health of all groups;

- Create social and physical environments that promote good health for all; and

- Promote quality of life, healthy development, and healthy behaviors across all life stages.

_____

_____

_____

_____

_____

_____

_____

Can Race Affect Health?

- The infant mortality rate is higher for African Americans.[6]
- Life expectancy is lower for African Americans.[7]
- African Americans have higher rates of hypertension.
- Native Americans have the highest diabetes rates.
- Caucasians have higher rates of osteoporosis, cystic fibrosis, skin cancer, and phenylketonuria (PKU).
- Chinese and Latina women have an increased risk of developing gestational diabetes.
- Asians metabolize some medications faster than whites.
- Ashkenazi Jews have higher rates of Tay-Sachs disease.[8]
- One in three Hispanics under the age of 65 has no health insurance.[9]

Factors Affecting Race and Health

- Genetics
- Environment
- Poverty
- Language barriers
- Unhealthy lifestyle
- Stress
- Illegal immigration status
- Income
- Education
- Discrimination

Can Gender Affect Health?[10]

- Women live longer than men.
- Women have higher rates of depression, panic attacks, arthritis, osteoporosis, and Alzheimer's disease.
- Women have higher rates of chronic diseases.
- Women score better on tests of verbal fluency.
- Women are more likely to be infected with a sexually transmitted disease (STD) during heterosexual contact.
- Women have a lower percentage of muscle.
- Women are more likely to attempt suicide.
- Men have higher rates of succeeding at suicide.
- Men are more prone to deadly diseases before age 50.
- Men suffer more injuries.
- Men score better in tests of visual-spatial ability.
- Men have higher rates of smoking and alcohol abuse.

How Healthy Is the U.S.?

- **Morbidity**—The relative incidence of disease.
- **Mortality**—The proportion of deaths to population.

During the 1900s, communicable diseases accounted for about 60 percent of all deaths. The top three causes of death in the United States in 1900 were:

1. Pneumonia/influenza,
2. Tuberculosis, and
3. Diarrhea/enteritis

These diseases were eradicated or nearly eliminated through better living conditions, hygiene, and the invention of antibiotics and vaccines. However, changes in living brought in other diseases, including lifestyle diseases. Since the 1940s, most deaths in the United States have resulted from lifestyle diseases such as heart disease, cancer, and strokes. And, by the late 1990s, lifestyle diseases accounted for more than 60 percent of all deaths. Certain forms of cancer, heart disease, high blood pressure, obesity, and Type 2 diabetes are lifestyle diseases because they are contracted from the way people live. Poor diet, lack of exercise, smoking, and excess alcohol and drug use, and poor sleep may contribute to these illnesses or be their primary cause. Researchers are saying that today's newborns may be the first generation to have a lower life expectancy than that of their parents. This is due to lifestyle risk factors, specifically obesity.

Examples of lifestyle diseases:

- Heart disease, "the #1 killer of both women and men," according to the National Institutes of Health, is most often caused by being overweight, not exercising, and smoking.
- Type 2 diabetes is when your body does not produce enough insulin or cannot use the insulin efficiently enough. This results in high blood sugar, since insulin is responsible for breaking down sugar to use for energy in the body. Diabetes can lead to long-term complications like kidney

disease, blindness, and poor wound healing. The lifestyle risk factors for diabetes include being overweight, not eating a healthy diet and physical inactivity.

- Among the most common infectious diseases are those that are sexually transmitted, with the Centers for Disease Control and Prevention reporting "19 million new STD infections each year . . ." Not using condoms is a lifestyle decision that predisposes one to fall victim to an STD or HIV/AIDS.

Though people are predisposed to many chronic illnesses because of genetics, age, gender or race, there are lifestyle changes you can make to decrease your chances of being affected. A person's health is his most precious asset. Good health allows you to fully participate in work and social activities. Your abilities become severely impaired when disease enters your life, whether it is for a short time or over an indefinite period. While anyone can become ill, there are strategies you can employ to help prevent disease. These include lifestyle changes geared toward protecting your health.

· ·

We are what we repeatedly do. Excellence, then, is not an act, but a habit.
—*Aristotle*

· ·

Habits and Your Health
· ·

A habit is an automatic behavior. The behavior has become automatic because it has been repeated frequently and thereby, turned over to subconscious control. We are all forming and reinforcing habits every day of our lives. Some are positive habits that move us toward our goals and some are negative that move us away from our goals. Any behavior that you repeat every day is habit-forming!

List your positive habits:

_____

_____

_____

_____

List your negative habits:

_____

_____

_____

_____

Most Harmful Personal Habits

1. Smoking
2. Drinking too much alcohol
3. Spending yourself into deep debt
4. Needing sleeping pills to get a good night's sleep
5. Taking painkillers every day

Most Harmful Lifestyle Choices

1. Being angry, worried, or stressed more than being happy
2. Not feeling in control
3. Being in an unhealthy relationship
4. Ignoring health signs and symptoms of disease
5. Not moving your body every day

Most Harmful Eating Habits

1. Drinking a lot of soda
2. Eating fast food more than 3 days/week
3. Skipping breakfast
4. Not eating vegetables daily
5. Yo-yo dieting

The Power of Positive Habits:
How to Change a Habit

1. Health Belief Model

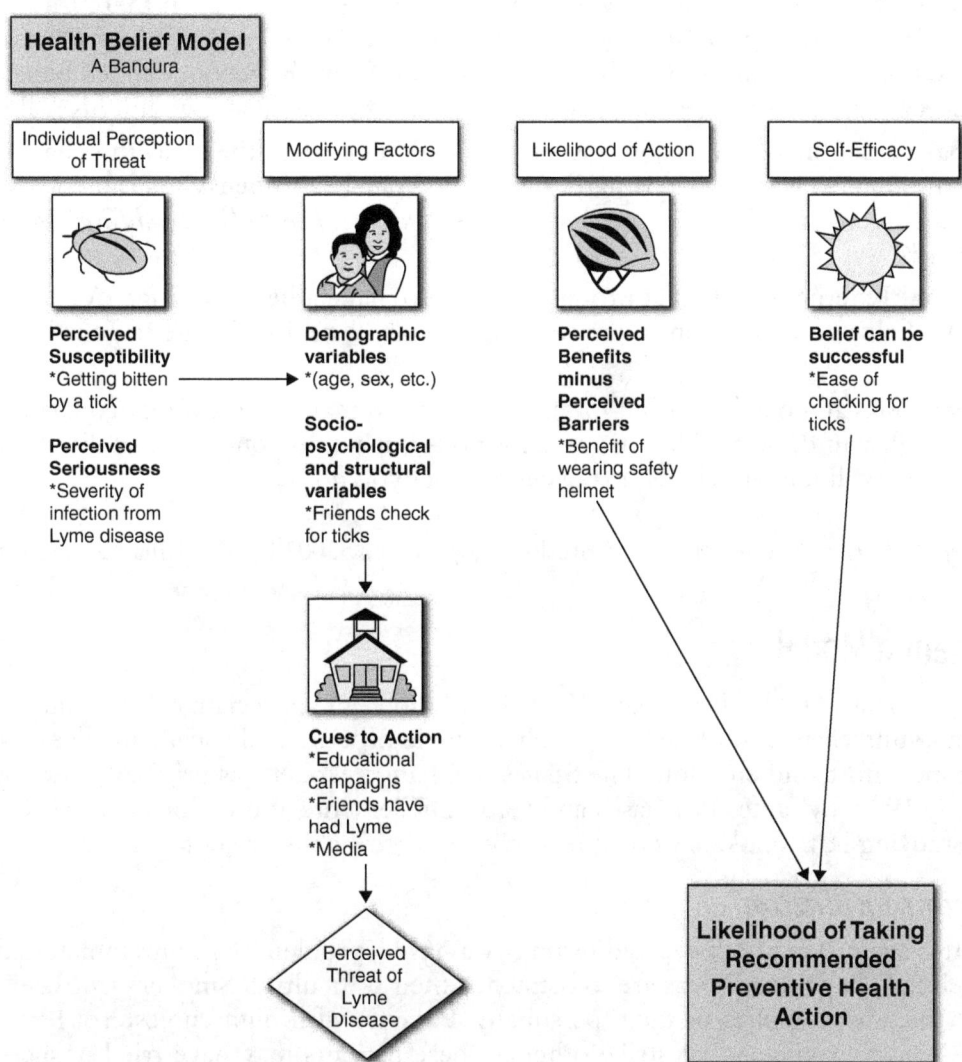

Source: Melanie Zibit MS, MBA, Medical Educator and Illustrator, Nancy Shadick, MD, MPH, and Brigham & Women's Hospital. Reproduced with permission.

The Health Belief Model (HBM) is a psychological model that attempts to explain and predict health behaviors. This is done by focusing on the attitudes and beliefs of individuals. The HBM was first developed in the 1950s by social psychologists Hochbaum, Rosenstock and Kegels working in the U.S. Public Health Services. The model was inspired by a study of why people sought X-ray examinations for tuberculosis. Since then, the HBM has been adapted to explore a variety of long- and short-term health behaviors, including sexual risk behaviors and the transmission of HIV/AIDS. The model postulates that the following six conditions both explain and predict a health-related behavior.

1. **Perceived Susceptibility**. A person believes that his or her health is in jeopardy. People will not change their health behaviors unless they believe that they are at risk. *Those who do not think that they are at risk of acquiring HIV from unprotected intercourse are unlikely to use a condom.*

2. **Perceived Severity**. The probability that a person will change his/her health behaviors to avoid a consequence depend on how serious he or she considers the consequence to be. The person perceives the "potential seriousness" of the condition in terms of pain or discomfort, time lost from work, economic difficulties, or other outcomes.

3. **Perceived Benefits**. It's difficult to convince people to change a behavior if there isn't something in it for them. *Your father stopped smoking because the doctor said his lungs are failing.* On assessing the circumstances, the person believes that benefits stemming from the recommended behavior outweigh the costs and inconvenience and that they are indeed possible and within his or her grasp.

4. **Perceived Barriers**. One of the major reasons people don't change their health behaviors is that they think that doing so is going to be hard. Changing your health behaviors can cost effort, money, and time. *If all your friends go out drinking on Saturdays, it may be very difficult to cut down on your alcohol intake.*

5. **Cues to Action**. External events that prompt a desire to make a health change. A cue to action is something that helps move someone from wanting to make a health change to actually making the change.

6. **Self-efficacy**. Looks at a person's belief in his/her ability to make a health related change. The belief in your ability to do something has an enormous impact on your actual ability to do it. Thinking that you will fail will almost make certain that you do.

From *Encyclopedia of Public Health* edited by Lester Breslow. Copyright © 2002 by MacMillan Reference USA.

2. Stages of Change Model

Anyone who has ever made and broken a New Year's Resolution can appreciate the difficulty of behavior change. Making a lasting change in behavior is rarely a simple process, and usually involves a substantial commitment of time, effort, and emotion. The Stages of Change Model was originally developed in the late 1970s and early 1980s by James Prochaska and Carlo DiClemente at the University of Rhode Island when they were studying how smokers were able to give up their habits or addiction.

Stage 1: Precontemplation

When you're at this stage, you aren't even admitting you have a problem. Precontemplators don't want to change themselves. They think others are to blame for their difficulties. Smokers who are "in denial" may not see that the advice applies to them personally. Patients with high cholesterol levels may feel "immune" to the health problems that strike others. Obese patients may have tried unsuccessfully so many times to lose weight that they have simply given up.

Stage 2: Contemplation

In this stage, you acknowledge you have a problem. You begin to think seriously about solving your problem. You start to assess barriers (e.g., time, expense, hassle, fear) as well as the benefits of change. You have indefinite plans to take action within the next few months.

Stage 3: Preparation

"If you fail to plan, you plan to fail."

You develop a detailed plan of action. You might be sampling low-fat foods or a move toward greater dietary modification, or decreasing your drinking.

Stage 4: Action

This stage is where you actually DO IT! You receive the most recognition and support during this stage, because others can see that you're working at it. You follow the plan you've made in Stage 3, making revisions as necessary.

Stage 5: Maintenance

The maintenance stage is a long, ongoing process, and for most people, it's the most difficult.

Celebrate achieving your goals, but don't relax just yet. Develop mental and behavioral coping strategies that will take you through the times when you feel you are beginning to slip.

Stage 6: Relapse

You must always maintain a life of vigilance. Some can progress to the point that they are not constantly tempted, nor do they think about it every day. Once you've had a deeply ingrained habit or addiction, you are always more vulnerable than if you'd never had it. Studies show that in times of stress or conflict, people are most likely to slip.

....

Habit is habit, and not to be flung out of the window by any man,
but coaxed downstairs a step at a time.

—*Mark Twain*

....

Steps to Change Unhealthy Behaviors

1. **Work on one habit at a time**. If you work on changing more than one habit at a time you run a serious risk of overwhelming yourself and changing no habits at all. To begin with, choose one unhealthy habit you wish to eliminate or change. Or, choose a healthy habit you want to adopt as part of your behavior. **It takes 21–30 days to break a bad habit.**

2. **Start small**. The smaller the better, because habit change is difficult, and trying to take on too much is a recipe for disaster. Want to exercise? Start with just 10–20 minutes.

3. **Create a plan and write it down**. Be as specific as possible. **Refine** your plan. Now you need to refine your plan. In particular, you need to be realistic. Put your plan in a drawer for a day or so and come back to it with fresh eyes. Make Mini-Plans (research psychologists call them "implementation intentions"). Write down all the details to make your big plan successful. For example, "when the alarm goes off at five, I will shower, get dressed, make a breakfast shake, and drive to work then at 5:30, I will eat a quick snack of yogurt and fruit and go to the gym." Researchers have shown the power of mini-plans to bridge the gap between wanting to get something done and getting it done. **Plan a support system**. Who will you turn to when you have a strong urge? Write these people into your plan. **Have rewards**. You might see these as bribes, but actually they're just positive feedback.

4. **Know your motivations, and be sure they're strong**. Write them down in your plan. You have to be very clear why you're doing this, and what the benefits are.

5. **Write down all your obstacles**. Write down every obstacle that's likely to happen. Then write down how you plan to overcome them. That's the key: write down your solution *before* the obstacles arrive, so you're prepared.

6. **Identify your triggers**. What situations trigger your current habit? For the smoking habit, for example, triggers might include going out with friends . . .

7. **For every single trigger, identify a positive habit you're going to do instead**. What will you do when you go out with friends, instead of smoking? What if someone offers you a cigarette? Some positive habits could include: exercise, meditation, deep breathing, and visualization.

8. **Become aware of self-talk**. Negative thoughts can derail any habit change. "I can't do this. This is too difficult. Why am I putting myself through this? How bad is this for me anyway?" It's important to take these negative thoughts and push them out of your head. Then replace them with a positive thought. "I can do this!"

9. **Plan strategies to defeat the negative urges**. Urges are going to come and go and they can be very strong and persuasive. But they're also temporary, and beatable. Urges usually last a few minutes, and they come in waves. You just need to ride out the wave, and the urge will go away. Some strategies for making it through the urge: deep breathing, self-massage, eat some frozen grapes, take a walk, exercise, drink a glass of water, call a support buddy, distract yourself.

10. **Use visualization**. This is a powerful tool. Vividly picture, in your head, successfully changing your habit. Visualize doing your new habit after each trigger, overcoming urges, and what it will look like when you're done.

11. **If you fail, figure out what went wrong, plan for it, and try again**. Don't let failure and guilt stop you. They're just obstacles, but they can be overcome. You should learn from each failure, and then they will become stepping stones to your success. When you fall off the horse, you have to get back on.

What Can You Do to Improve Your Health?

- Wear a seat belt.
- Stop smoking, binge-drinking, and abusing drugs.
- Exercise.
- Cut down on fast food.
- Cut down on caffeine.
- Reach your ideal body weight.
- Drink eight glasses of water every day.
- Perform regular body self-exams.
- Take regular stress breaks.
- Get enough sleep.
- Eat your fruits and vegetables.
- Volunteer.
- Be kind to yourself and to others.

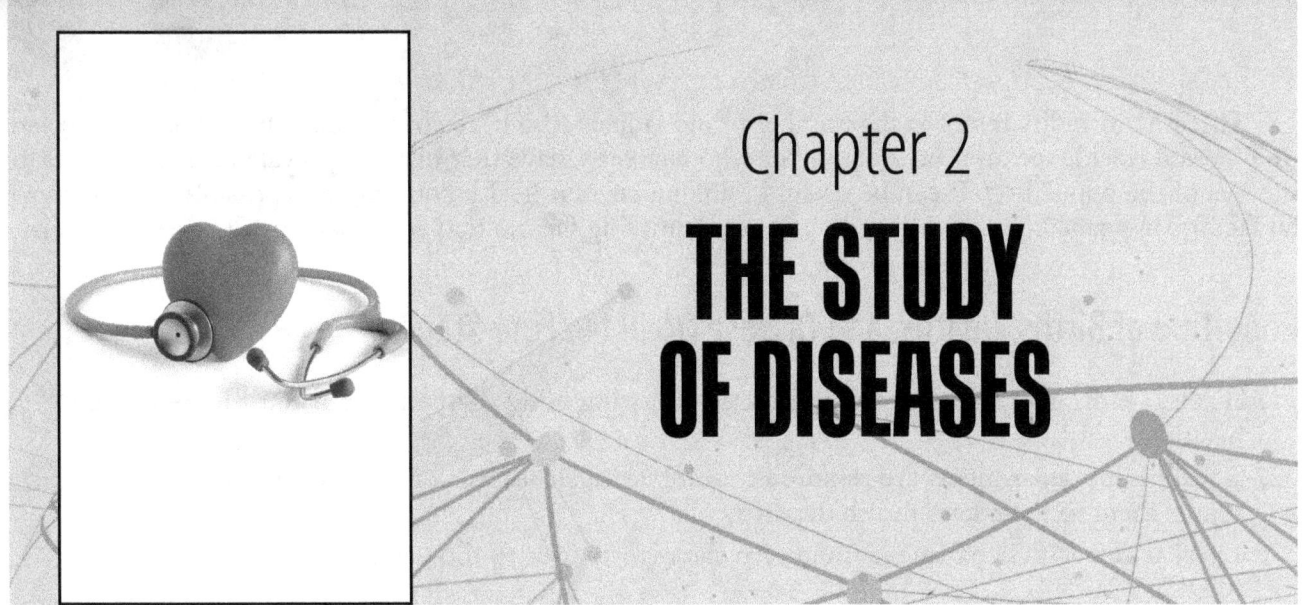

Chapter 2
THE STUDY OF DISEASES

Every human being is the author of his own health or disease.
—*Hindu Prince Guatama Siddhartha, Founder of Buddahism*

Nearly everywhere around the world, people are living longer but increasingly; people are battling with the diseases and disabilities of modern life.

Community health education is designed to promote health and prevent disease within populations. People who study community health use their knowledge to develop and implement programs that are intended to maintain health and prevent diseases to the extent possible for specific populations in a community.

Much of the work of community health revolves around three basic tools: epidemiology, community organizing, and health education.

Epidemiology

Epidemiology is a branch of medicine that involves the study of the causes, distribution, and control of disease in populations. Its focus is on the factors that affect both the health and illness of populations.

An **epidemiologist** might work on a wide range of issues, including investigations related to outbreaks of diseases and environmental exposure to toxins; the general promotion of health; and the development of biological, statistical, (en.wikipedia.org) and psychosocial theories regarding disease. Important aspects of the work of epidemiologists include identifying and defining diseases, making causational connections between and among diseases, and formulating effective strategies for health.

Disease Mortality versus Disease Morbidity

Disease mortality is a measure of the number of deaths in a population. Reporting deaths is a legal requirement supported by a national collection system. A sudden increase in deaths due to identical causes in one geographic region can alert health officials to an environmental problem, such as a waterborne disease outbreak.

Disease morbidity refers to the number of individuals who have contracted a disease during a given time period (incidence rate) or the number who currently have that disease (prevalence rate), scaled to the size of the population. It can be useful in linking current health conditions to possible environmental factors, in analyzing disease trends, and/or identifying factors that cause specific diseases or trends.

Reporting of Births, Deaths, and Disease Occurs in Four Steps:

1. Births, deaths, and cases of certain diseases occurring in the United States, must be reported to health authorities.
2. Local health departments are required to summarize all records of birth, deaths, and diseases and report them to their state health departments.
3. Local state health departments then turn the reports over to the Centers for Disease Control (CDC).
4. Local, state, and federal governments maintain vital and disease records that are used by health professionals to track and study disease.

Factors Affecting a Country's Mortality Rate

- Age of country's population
- Nutrition levels
- Standards of diet and housing
- Access to clean drinking water
- Hygiene levels
- Levels of infectious diseases
- Levels of violent crime
- Conflicts
- Number of doctors

Infant Mortality Rate

Infant mortality and life expectancy are two key indicators of any nation's overall health. **Infant mortality** is the death of infants in the first year of life. Major causes of infant mortality in more developed countries include infection and sudden infant death syndrome (SIDS). U.S. rates are still higher than those of other developed countries. The most common cause of infant mortality of all children around the world is pneumonia, dehydration from diarrhea, and malnutrition due to poverty, and unsafe food and water.

U.S. Infant Mortality Among Worst in Industrialized Nations

Among 33 industrialized nations, the United States is tied with Hungary, Malta, Poland, and Slovakia with a death rate of nearly 5 per 1,000 babies. Japan had the lowest newborn death rate, 1.8 per 1,000.

The high infant mortality in U.S. is driven partly by racial and income healthcare disparities. In the United States the population is more racially and economically diverse than many other industrialized countries, making it more challenging to provide culturally appropriate healthcare. Among African Americans, there are 9 deaths per 1,000 live births, closer to rates in developing nations than to those in the industrialized world. About half a million U.S. babies are born prematurely each year. African-American babies are twice as likely as white infants to be premature, to have a low birth weight, and to die at birth.

Possible factors that contribute to the low U.S. rankings include:

- High rates of teen pregnancies
- High obesity rates
- Lack of a free universal health insurance
- Short maternal maternity leave
- Poor access to healthcare
- Poverty and discrimination

Those factors can lead to poor healthcare before and during pregnancy, increasing risks for premature births and low birth weight, which are the leading causes of newborn death in industrialized countries. The impoverished nations account for 99 percent of the 4 million annual deaths of babies in their first month. The highest rates globally were in Africa and South Asia. Infections are the main culprit.

Classification of Diseases and Health Problems

Diseases and health problems can be classified in several meaningful ways.

A **communicable disease** is an infectious disease that is capable of being transmitted from one person or species to another (en.wikipedia.org). Communicable diseases are spread through direct contact with an infected individual or contact with bodily fluids or objects of infected individuals.

An **infectious disease** is a disease of humans or animals that damages or injures the host. This type of disease results from the presence of microbial agents that include: viruses, bacteria, fungi, protozoa, multicellular parasites, and prions (aberrant proteins). Poor people, women, children, and the elderly are the most vulnerable. Infectious diseases continue to be the world's leading killer of young adults and children.

- **Infectivity**—the ability of an organism to enter, survive, and multiply in the host.
- **Infectiousness**—the ease with which the disease is transmitted to other hosts (en.wikipedia.org).

An **infection** is different than an infectious disease because an infection may not cause clinical symptoms or impair host function.

The World Health Organization collects information on global deaths by International Classification of Disease (ICD) code categories.

Top Infectious Diseases Globally

Lower respiratory infections
1. HIV/AIDS
2. Diarrheal diseases

3. Tuberculosis (TB)

4. Malaria

5. Measles

6. Pertussis

7. Tetanus

8. Meningitis

9. Syphilis

(Source: World Health Organization at www.who.int/whosis/icd10/)

How Infections Spread

The chain of infection is a model that conceptualizes the transmission of a communicable disease from its source to a new susceptible host. Each link must be present and in sequential order for an infection to occur. The links are: infectious agent, reservoir, portal of exit from the reservoir, mode of transmission, and portal of entry into a susceptible host. An awareness of this cycle also provides knowledge of methods of self-protection.

An **infectious agent** is a microbial organism that can cause disease. Infectious agents include bacteria, virus, fungi, and parasites.

- **Bacteria:** Bacteria are unicellular organisms. They multiply by dividing themselves into new bacteria. Bacteria exist everywhere, including inside and on humans' bodies. Some bacteria live in the intestines and help boost the immune system. These are referred to as "good" bacteria. To maintain a healthy level of good bacteria, people must take in probiotics or eat yogurt that contains active live cultures. On the other hand, people sometimes need to take antibiotics to kill harmful bacteria. However, antibiotics kill not only the bad bacteria, but also the good bacteria. The overuse of antibiotics has caused bacteria today to be more resistant to these drugs and renders them more difficult to kill.

- **Viruses:** Unlike bacteria, viruses cannot multiply by themselves, so they must invade a host cell and take over its function to be able to create new viral cells. Viruses are made of genetic material (DNA or RNA) surrounded by a protective protein coat. Viruses can invade cells, and once they do, they take over the cells and reproduce new viral cells. The host cells usually die after the reproduction of new viral cells. RNA viruses are unstable and thus often mutate, whereas DNA viruses are more stable and mutate less often.

  Antibiotics are ineffective against viruses, such as colds and flu. Thus, it is important for people to limit the use of antibiotics only to bacterial infections. Again, the overuse of antibiotics decreases their effectiveness by encouraging the growth of antibiotic-resistant bacteria, which has become an increasingly serious worldwide problem.

A **reservoir** is a place in which microorganisms live and reproduce. Microorganisms thrive within the bodies of humans and animals, as well as in water and on tabletops and doorknobs.

A **portal of entry** is an opening in which a microorganism is able to enter the body of a host. Some portals of entry include body orifices, mucus membranes, and cuts in the skin.

A **susceptible host** is a body that a microorganism can invade, multiply, and cause an infection.

A **portal of exit** is a place from which microorganisms leave a reservoir. An example of a microorganism leaving a portal of exit is when they are expelled through the nose or mouth when a person sneezes or coughs.

A **mode of transmission** is a method by which an organism travels from one infected individual or group to an uninfected individual or group. Modes of transmission can be direct or indirect. **Direct transmission** includes touching (including through sexual contact), coughing, and sneezing. **Indirect transmission** can be airborne, vehicle-borne, or vector-borne.

The following are definitions of different modes of disease transmission:

- **Droplet contact:** coughing or sneezing on another person.
- **Direct physical contact:** touching an infected person, including sexual contact.
- **Indirect contact:** touching a contaminated surface, including, in some cases, soil.
- **Airborne transmission:** occurs when a microorganism can remain in the air for a long period of time.
- **Fecal-oral transmission:** often occurs from contaminated food or water sources.
- **Vector-borne transmission:** the carrying of disease by insects or other animals.

The Role of Humans in the Transmission of Diseases

The construction of new housing developments in previously uninhabited areas brings people into contact with animals and thus with the microbes that they harbor as well. In Florida, for example, many swamplands are being destroyed to make way for new construction of homes. But the alligators, as well as the microbes associated with them, remain in the vicinity, and eventually these microbes can be transmitted to people. This type of disease transmission also occurs in the rain forests that are being cut down.

Disease transmission to and by humans also results when the rapid growth of cities, particularly in developing countries, forces large numbers of people into crowded areas with poor sanitation. In addition, global warming changes ecosystems in ways that move microbes into new areas.

Disease Control

A major goal of public health is to prevent the spread of infectious diseases in populations and to contain outbreaks when they do occur. Vaccines are a primary means of preventing diseases in people who receive them. Vaccines prevent and control many infectious diseases that were once common in the United States, including polio, mumps, measles, diphtheria, tetanus, pertussis (whooping cough), rubella (German measles), and *Haemophilus influenzae type* b (Hib).

(Source: Centers for Disease Control)

What is a vaccine?

A vaccine exposes a person to germs in a safe manner. A vaccine contains dead or weakened germs that cause a specific type of disease. When a person is vaccinated, his or her body reacts by creating protective substances called antibodies, which defend the body by helping to kill the germs that enter the body. The person does not contract the particular disease but is then protected from it.

Like a real disease, a vaccine creates **active immunity** because the body has a lasting memory of the infection. **Passive immunity** is acquired through breast milk or immunoglobulin shots given for allergies. Passive immunity lasts for only a few months. **Herd immunity** is the protection not just of a vaccinated person but also of others who come in contact with that person. Through herd immunity, it is sometimes possible to completely **eradicate** an infection, which occurs when there is no risk of infection or disease anywhere in the world. So far, the only infectious disease that has been eradicated is smallpox, the last case of which occurred in 1979. However, because several laboratories kept samples of the smallpox virus, it is not actually extinct. **Extinction** occurs when an agent no longer exists in nature or in a laboratory.

Disease Prevention, Control, and Intervention

Prevention is taking action to avert the onset of a disease before it is contracted. **Intervention** is taking action to control a disease in progress.

Control is the containment of a disease and can include both prevention and intervention. Prevention is clearly the best means of controlling a disease.

Levels of Prevention

- **Primary prevention** is averting an illness before the disease process can begin (e.g., education).
- **Secondary prevention** is the early diagnosis and immediate treatment of a disease before it becomes advanced and disability becomes severe (e.g., screening).
- **Tertiary prevention** is the retraining, reeducating, and rehabilitating of a person who has already contracted and is suffering from a disease (e.g., emergency medical services).

Breaking the Cycle of Infection

Preventing infection is a matter of examining one's lifestyle choices, habits, and environment, and then assessing which of these areas might lead to infection. By identifying areas in the chain of infection, people can take steps to eliminate them. The following are some basic steps to help prevent infections:

- Practice good personal hygiene. Frequent and proper hand washing is essential in preventing the spread of infection.
  - Always wash your hands with regular soap while singing the entire happy birthday song.
- Treat all bodily fluids as potentially infectious.
  - Use protective barriers such as gloves, masks, aprons, and condoms when exposure to infectious agents is possible.
- Maintain a clean home and environment.
- Store and cook foods at the proper temperatures.
- Properly dispose of wastes, garbage, and used medical supplies.
- See your doctor regularly for protective vaccines and immunizations.

Communicable versus Noncommunicable Diseases

Noncommunicable diseases cannot be transmitted from one person to another. For example, diseases of the heart and blood vessels are noncommunicable diseases. They are the leading cause of death in the United States.

Communicable diseases are infectious diseases that can be transmitted from an infected person to another, either by direct contact or indirectly.

Example of Communicable Diseases

Human Influenza (Flu)

Influenza, or the flu, is a contagious respiratory illness caused by influenza viruses. The flu is associated with mild to severe symptoms and illness. It some cases, it can cause death. Every year, between 5 percent and 20 percent of the population of the United States contracts the flu. Some people, such as older people, young children, and people with certain health conditions are at a higher risk for serious flu complications, which can include bacterial pneumonia, ear infections, sinus infections, dehydration, and worsening of chronic medical conditions, such as congestive heart failure, asthma, and diabetes. Today, about 250,000 to 500,000 people worldwide die of influenza every year (cdc.gov/flu).

A **flu epidemic** occurs when a flu virus spreads rapidly throughout a population. Flu epidemics are common within certain populations nearly every year. In contrast, an **influenza pandemic** is an epidemic of an influenza virus that spreads throughout the world and infects a large percentage of the human population. Unlike the common seasonal epidemics of influenza, pandemics do not occur as often.

Based on historical records, influenza pandemics have most likely occurred during at least the last four centuries. Since the early 1900s, three pandemics and several "pandemic threats" have occurred.

Symptoms of flu include the following:

- Fever
- Headache
- Extreme tiredness
- Dry cough
- Sore throat
- Runny or stuffy nose
- Muscle aches
- Stomach symptoms, such as nausea, vomiting, and diarrhea, also can occur, but these are more common in children than adults.

Flu viruses typically spread from one person to another through the coughing or sneezing of a person who has influenza or by touching something with a flu virus on it and then touching the mouth or nose. Healthy adults often are able to infect others beginning just one day before symptoms develop and up to five days after becoming ill.

Treatment and Prevention

Prevention is key by making sure your immune system stays healthy. Eating healthy fruit and vegetables, avoiding sugar, fat, and chemicals in your food will increase your killer cells (T-cells) to fight off the virus. Washing your hands regularly with plain soap is a key prevention strategy. If you do get the flu, drink many fluids, get plenty of rest, and make sure you are getting immune boosting vitamins like Vitamin D3 and Vitamin C from your diet.

The **flu shot** is an inactivated vaccine, meaning that it contains the dead virus. The flu shot is approved for people age 6 months and older, both for those who are healthy and those who have chronic medical conditions. About two weeks after receiving the flu shot, a person's body develops antibodies that protect against an influenza virus infection.

Another form of a vaccination for influenza is in the form of a nasal spray (cdc.gov/flu). The nasal-spray flu vaccine, sometimes called LAIV for "Live Attenuated Influenza Vaccine," is made with a live, weakened flu virus. The LAIV is approved for use in healthy people 5 to 49 years of age who are not pregnant.

People at high risk for complications from the flu include the following:

- Children age 6 months to 5 years
- Pregnant women
- People 50 years of age and older
- People of any age with certain chronic medical conditions, such as asthma
- Healthcare workers
- People who live in nursing homes and other long-term care facilities

The Pandemic of Lifestyle Diseases

In the early 1900s, the leading causes of death in the United States were communicable diseases such as pneumonia, influenza, tuberculosis, and diarrhea. Since the 1940s, however, the majority of deaths in the United States have resulted from diseases related to lifestyles, such as heart disease, obesity, diabetes, hypertension, stroke, and cancer.

Lifestyle diseases are those that result from the ways in which people live: diet, habits, environment, and levels of exercise all play critical roles in the development or non-development of such diseases. Lifestyle diseases are different from other diseases because they are potentially preventable, and the risk of contracting them can be reduced by an awareness in and appropriate changes in diet, lifestyle, habits, and environment.

Many lifestyle diseases are related to obesity and physical inactivity. These include heart disease, type 2 diabetes, hypertension, atherosclerosis, asthma, cancer, chronic liver disease or cirrhosis of the liver, chronic obstructive pulmonary disease, metabolic syndrome, nephritis or chronic renal failure, osteoporosis, stroke, and depression.

Chronic Lifestyle Diseases

Heart Disease

Cardiovascular diseases (CVDs) rank as America's number-one killer, claiming the lives of nearly 38 percent of the more than 2.4 million Americans who die each year. Approximately 70.1 million Americans have some type of cardiovascular disease. Cancer follows in severity, killing about 23 percent of those who die each year.[56] Someone dies of heart disease every 35 seconds in the United States.

What Is Coronary Artery Disease?

Coronary artery disease is caused by a narrowing or blocking of the blood vessels that go to your heart. It's the most common form of heart disease. Your blood carries oxygen and other needed materials to your heart. Blood vessels to your heart can become partially or totally blocked by fatty deposits. A heart attack occurs when the blood supply to your heart is reduced or cut off.

Risk Factors for Cardiovascular Disease

Factors You Can Control

Lifestyle factors contribute to the majority of CVD cases in the United States:

- Physical inactivity
- Tobacco use
- Obesity
- Blood fats
- Metabolic syndrome
- Diabetes mellitus

Factors You Can't Control

- Heredity
- Race and ethnicity
- Age
- Gender
- Bacterial infection

Factors

The following nine risk factors account for 90 percent of heart disease diagnosis:[57]

1. **Abdominal obesity** more than doubles heart attack risk in both men and women. Abdominal fat is hormonally active.

2. **Alcohol** acts as a platelet blocker. Modest amounts of alcohol (one or more drinks) reduce a man's heart attack risk by 12 percent and a woman's by 60 percent. Wine has been shown to be highest in protective antioxidants. Too much beer or hard liquor, more than a drink a day, can promote heart disease, cancer, and alcoholism.

3. **Bad cholesterol**—high cholesterol roughly quadruples heart attack risk. It works this way: Bad cholesterol (LDL) carries fats into the artery wall; good cholesterol (HDL) carts it away. A sedentary lifestyle and fatty diet increase LDL and lower HDL. Exercise and a healthy diet switch that ratio and keep arteries clear.

4. **Diabetes** is especially deadly for women, quadrupling their risk of having a heart attack. Men with diabetes double their risk of a heart attack. Like smoking, diabetes causes platelets to stick together, resulting in tiny clots. These clots clog the microscopic blood vessels that feed nerves and arteries, which is a key reason diabetes destroys circulation. Diabetes also raises the level of harmful fats in the blood.

5. **Not eating fruits and vegetables**—eating fruits and vegetables daily cuts heart risk by 30 to 40 percent. Fruits and vegetables lower bad cholesterol, improve blood sugar, and replace foods that might not be as healthy.

6. **Sedentary lifestyle**—moderate exercise reduces a man's heart risk by 23 percent and a woman's by twice that amount. Exercise improves cholesterol, staves off diabetes by improving blood sugar, and promotes blood vessel growth.

7. **High blood pressure** nearly triples a man's risk of having a heart attack and more than doubles a woman's. Narrowed blood vessels force the heart to work harder, slowly wearing it out. The blood's friction against artery walls also can promote the rupture of plaques, which can lead to heart attacks.

8. **Psychosocial stress**—stressful life events, behavioral disorders, and depression nearly triple heart attack risk. Depressed people with heart disease are four times more likely to have a heart attack or die, and depression is prevalent among 20 percent of people with heart disease in the United States.

9. **Smoking**—smokers are two to three times more likely to have a heart attack than people who don't smoke. Cigarette smoke damages the artery wall, paving the way for inflammation and cholesterol buildup. It narrows arteries. It also activates platelets, sticky cells that cling together and promote clotting. When cholesterol deposits burst inside arteries, clots form.

From USA TODAY, a division of Gannett Co., Inc. Reprinted by Permission.

Facts About Women and Cardiovascular Disease[58]

Misperceptions still exist that CVD is not a real problem for women.

- Cardiovascular disease claims more women's lives than the next six causes of death combined—about 500,000 women's lives a year.
- CVD is a particularly important problem among minority women. The death rate due to CVD is substantially higher in black women than in white women.
- 38 percent of women compared with 25 percent of men will die within one year after a heart attack.
- More women than men die of stroke.
- Low blood levels of good cholesterol (high-density lipoprotein, or HDL) appear to be a stronger predictor of heart disease death in women than in men in the over-65 age group; high blood levels of triglycerides (another type of fat) may be a particularly important risk factor in women and the elderly.
- Diagnosis of heart disease presents a greater challenge in women than in men.
- Women's symptoms are underrecognized, misinterpreted, and sometimes different than men's.
- An apple body shape is more dangerous than a pear shape.
- A sedentary lifestyle contributes to CVD risk.
- Women's heartbeats are faster, thus it takes longer to relax.

How the Heart Works

The normal heart is a strong, hard-working pump made of muscle tissue. It's about the size of a person's fist.

The heart has four chambers. The upper two chambers are the right atrium and left atrium, and the lower two are the right ventricle and left ventricle. Blood is pumped through the chambers, aided by four heart valves. The valves open and close to let the blood flow in only one direction.

The four heart valves are:

1. Tricuspid valve, located between the right atrium and the right ventricle.
2. Pulmonary (pulmonic) valve, between the right ventricle and the pulmonary artery.
3. Mitral valve, between the left atrium and left ventricle.
4. Aortic valve, between the left ventricle and the aorta.

Dark bluish blood, low in oxygen, flows back to the heart after circulating through the body. It returns to the heart through veins and enters the right atrium. This chamber empties blood through the tricuspid valve into the right ventricle. The right ventricle pumps the blood under low pressure through the pulmonary valve into the pulmonary artery. From there the blood goes to the lungs, where it gets fresh oxygen. After the blood is refreshed with oxygen, it is bright red. Then it returns by the pulmonary veins to the left atrium. From there it passes through the mitral valve and enters the left ventricle.

The left ventricle pumps the red oxygen-rich blood out through the aortic valve into the aorta. The aorta takes blood to the body's general circulation. The blood pressure in the left ventricle is the same as the pressure measured in the arm.

What Do Your Cholesterol Numbers Mean?

Everyone age 20 and older should have their cholesterol measured at least once every five years. It is best to have a blood test called a *lipoprotein profile* to find out your cholesterol numbers. This blood test should be done after a 9- to 12-hour fast and gives information about your:

- Total cholesterol
- LDL (bad) cholesterol—the main source of cholesterol buildup and blockage in the arteries
- HDL (good) cholesterol—helps keep cholesterol from building up in the arteries
- Triglycerides—free-floating fatty acids in your blood

What Affects Cholesterol Levels?

- **Diet.** Saturated fat and cholesterol in the food you eat make your blood cholesterol level go up. Reducing the amount of saturated fat and cholesterol in your diet helps lower your blood cholesterol level.

  Foods to avoid for high cholesterol/high triglycerides:
  - Full-fat dairy
  - Fatty meats
  - Tropical oils
  - Trans-fats
  - Simple sugars

Total Cholesterol Level	Category
Less than 200 mg/dL	Desirable
200–239 mg/dL	Borderline high
240 mg/dL and above	High
LDL Cholesterol Level	**Category**
Less than 100 mg/dL	Optimal
HDL Cholesterol Level	**Category**
Greater than 60 mg/dL	Optimal
Triglyceride Level	**Category**
Less than 150 mg/dL	Optimal

Foods to include:

- High-fiber/whole grains
- Fruits/vegetables
- Nuts
- Legumes

- **Weight.** BMI >25 means you are overweight. Being overweight is a major risk factor for heart disease. It also tends to increase your cholesterol. Losing weight if you are overweight can help lower LDL and is especially important for those with a cluster of risk factors that includes high triglyceride and/or low HDL levels and being overweight with a large waist measurement (more than 40 inches for men and more than 35 inches for women).
- **Physical activity.** Not being physically active is a major risk factor for heart disease. Regular physical activity can help lower LDL (bad) cholesterol and triglycerides, and raise HDL (good) cholesterol levels. It also helps you lose weight. You should try to be physically active for at least 30 minutes on most if not all days.

Things you cannot do anything about also can affect your cholesterol levels. These include:

- **Age and gender.** As women and men get older, their cholesterol levels rise. Before the age of menopause, women have lower total cholesterol levels than men of the same age. After the age of menopause, women's LDL levels tend to rise.
- **Heredity.** Your genes partly determine how much cholesterol your body makes. High blood cholesterol can run in families.

Heart Attack Warning Signs[59]

Some heart attacks are sudden and intense—the "movie heart attack"—where no one doubts what's happening. But most heart attacks start slowly, with mild pain or discomfort. Often people affected aren't sure what's wrong and wait too long before getting help.

- **Chest discomfort.** Most heart attacks involve discomfort in the center of the chest that lasts more than a few minutes, or that goes away and comes back. It can feel like uncomfortable pressure, squeezing, fullness, or pain.
- **Discomfort in other areas of the upper body.** Symptoms can include pain or discomfort in one or both arms, the back, neck, jaw, or stomach.
- **Shortness of breath.** May occur with or without chest discomfort.
- **Other signs.** These may include breaking out in a cold sweat, nausea, or lightheadedness.

As with men, women's most common heart attack symptom is chest pain or discomfort. But women are somewhat more likely than men to experience some of the other common symptoms, particularly shortness of breath, nausea/vomiting, and back, abdominal, or jaw pain.

If you or someone you're with has chest discomfort, especially with one or more of the other signs, don't wait longer than a few minutes (no more than five) before calling for help. **Call 911.** Get to a hospital right away.

Smoking and Heart Disease

- Smoking is the single most significant risk factor for CV disease and peripheral vascular disease.
- Each year smoking causes 250,000+ deaths from cardiovascular disease.
- Active and passive smoking are both detrimental.

How Smoking Damages the Heart
- Nicotine overstimulates the heart.
- Carbon monoxide reduces the oxygen supply to the heart.
- Tars and other smoke residues increase the risk of cholesterol buildup in the arteries.
- Smoking increases blood clotting.
- Smoking causes irreversible damage to the arteries.

What Is a Stroke?

A stroke occurs when the blood supply to a portion of the brain is blocked. Strokes are the third-leading cause of death in the United States.

Risk Factors for Strokes
- Gender
- Race
- Age
- Hypertension
- High red blood cell count
- Heart disease
- Blood fats
- Diabetes mellitus

Warning Signs of Strokes
- Sudden numbness or weakness of the face, arm, or leg—particularly on one side of the body
- Sudden confusion, difficulty in speech or understanding
- Sudden trouble seeing out of one or both eyes
- Sudden trouble walking, dizziness, loss of balance or coordination
- A sudden, severe headache of unknown cause

Diabetes

Diabetes is a serious illness that is increasing rapidly in New York City and around the country. In just the past eight years, the number of New Yorkers with diabetes has doubled. Diabetes is reaching epidemic numbers.[60,61]

- An estimated 800,000 adult New Yorkers—more than one in every eight—now have diabetes.
- Thousands of New Yorkers have dangerous diabetes-related complications.
- New York, perhaps more than any other big city, harbors all the ingredients for a continued epidemic. It has large numbers of poor and obese citizens, who are at higher risk. It has a growing population of Latinos, who get the disease in disproportionate numbers, and of Asians, who can develop it at much lower weights than people of other races.

- One in three children born in the United States in the year 2000 are expected to become diabetic in their lifetimes, according to a projection by the Centers for Disease Control and Prevention. The forecast is even bleaker for Latinos: one in every two.
- Diabetics are two to four times more likely than others to develop heart disease or have a stroke, and three times more likely to die of complications from pneumonia. Most diabetics suffer nervous-system damage and poor circulation, which can lead to amputations of toes, feet, and entire legs; even a tiny cut on the foot can lead to gangrene because it will not be seen or felt.
- Women with diabetes are at higher risk for complications in pregnancy, including miscarriages and birth defects. Men run a higher risk of impotence. Young adults have twice the chance of getting gum disease and losing teeth.

What Is Diabetes?

Diabetes is a disease in which the body does not produce or properly use insulin. Insulin is a hormone that is needed to convert sugar, starches, and other food into energy needed for daily life. The cause of diabetes continues to be a mystery, although both genetics and environmental factors such as obesity and lack of exercise appear to play roles.

Diabetes Causes Serious Health Problems

- Heart disease and atherosclerosis (hardening of the arteries)
- Stroke
- Eye problems and blindness
- Kidney disease
- Poor circulation
- Nerve damage
- Foot and leg problems, which can lead to amputation
- Skin problems (infections, boils, scaly skin, itching)
- Gum disease and other oral health problems
- Erectile dysfunction (impotence) in men
- Depression
- Premature death

Diabetes Often Has No Symptoms

Many people with diabetes have no symptoms, symptoms that develop gradually over months or even years, or symptoms so mild they go unnoticed. Possible symptoms include:

- Frequent urination
- Excessive thirst and hunger
- Weight loss
- Weakness and fatigue
- Nausea and vomiting
- Sudden vision changes
- Tingling or numbness in hands or feet
- Frequent or slow-healing sores or infections
- Recurring vaginal yeast infections in women

Major Types of Diabetes[62]

Type 1 Diabetes

Cause: results from the body's failure to produce insulin, the hormone that unlocks the cells of the body, allowing glucose to enter and fuel them. It is estimated that 5 to 10 percent of Americans who are diagnosed with diabetes have type 1 diabetes. The immune system attacks cells in the pancreas, preventing the production of insulin.

Age of onset: as early as infancy.

Physical condition: normal weight or thin.

Treatment: insulin injections or pump; close monitoring of blood sugar.

Type 2 Diabetes

Cause: results from insulin resistance (a condition in which the body fails to properly use insulin), combined with relative insulin deficiency. Obesity, resulting from an unhealthy diet and lack of exercise, makes cells resistant to insulin. Most Americans who are diagnosed with diabetes have type 2 diabetes. *Overweight and obesity are the biggest risk factors for type 2 diabetes.*

Risk factors for type 2 diabetes include:

- Overweight and obesity
- Lack of physical activity
- Older age
- Family history of diabetes, or prior gestational diabetes
- Low levels of HDL ("good") cholesterol or high levels of triglycerides (fats) in the blood
- Race/ethnicity—African Americans, Latinos, Native Americans, and some Asian Americans and Pacific Islanders are at higher risk

Age of onset: as early as age 6, but typically age 10 and up.

Physical condition: typically overweight or obese.

Treatment: dietary changes; increased exercise; blood-sugar-lowering medication.

Gestational Diabetes (Pregnancy-related)

Gestational diabetes affects about 4 to 7 percent of all pregnant women. About half of these women will develop type 2 diabetes within 10 years. If untreated or poorly controlled, gestational diabetes can harm a developing baby.

Pre-Diabetes

Pre-diabetes is a condition that occurs when a person's blood glucose levels are higher than normal but not high enough for a diagnosis of type 2 diabetes. There are 41 million Americans who have pre-diabetes, in addition to the 20.8 million with diabetes. People with pre-diabetes are 50 percent more likely to have a heart attack or stroke. Unless they take steps to control weight and increase physical activity, most people with pre-diabetes will develop type 2 diabetes.

Prevention of Diabetes (Type 2)

- Maintain a healthy weight. If you are overweight or obese, lose at least 5 to 10 percent of body weight.
- Get at least 30 minutes of moderate physical activity (such as a brisk walk) on all or most days.

- Eat a diet high in fiber, fruits, and vegetables, and low in saturated fats.
- These lifestyle changes can lower the risk of developing type 2 diabetes by up to 60 percent in people at risk.

To Manage Diabetes, Know Your "ABC'S"

People with diabetes can prevent heart and kidney disease, blindness, amputations, and other complications by knowing and controlling their "ABC'S":

- **A**1C (three-month average blood sugar level): *Less than 7 percent.*
- **B**lood pressure: *Less than 130/80.*
- **C**holesterol: *LDL ("bad") cholesterol less than 100.*
- **S**moking: *If you smoke, quit now. (For free help, call the Smokers' Quit Line at 311.)*

Hypertension

Hypertension is known as the silent killer. One in four adult New Yorkers have been told they have high blood pressure. Hundreds of thousands more have it *but don't know it*. It causes the heart to pump harder than normal and wears out the arteries. The pressure of blood against the walls of arteries is recorded as two numbers: the systolic pressure (as the heart beats) over the diastolic pressure (as the heart relaxes between beats). Normal blood pressure is less than 120 milliliters of mercury systolic and less than 80 milliliters mercury diastolic.

Systolic blood pressure (top number): Pressure exerted by blood against the walls of the arteries during forceful *contraction* of the heart.

Diastolic blood pressure (bottom number): Pressure exerted by blood against the walls of the arteries during *relaxation* of the heart.

Nearly 50 million Americans have high blood pressure. If left untreated, high blood pressure can lead to strokes, heart attacks, and kidney failure. Conversely, controlling elevated blood pressure can cut strokes 35 to 40 percent and heart attacks 20 to 25 percent. Often, dietary and other lifestyle changes are sufficient to keep blood pressure controlled. If not, it may be necessary to add blood pressure medications such as diuretics, ACE inhibitors, beta blockers, or calcium channel blockers.[63] African Americans are more likely than other groups to have high blood pressure.

Why High Blood Pressure Is Dangerous[64]

- High blood pressure means the force of blood is too strong.
- This makes the heart work harder, which causes the muscle to become thick and stiff.
- It also damages blood vessels, which makes it easier for cholesterol and other substances to build up.
- Untreated high blood pressure increases the risk of:
  - Heart disease
  - Stroke
  - Problems with blood vessels and circulation
  - Kidney and eye problems
  - Premature death

Preventing High Blood Pressure

- Lifestyle changes
- Losing weight
- Regular exercise
- Dietary approaches to stop hypertension (DASH diet)
- Restriction of daily sodium intake
- Quit smoking—nicotine raises blood pressure and heart rate. If you have high blood pressure and smoke, you more than double your risk of a heart attack.

What Can I Do to Prevent Chronic Diseases?

Making wise food choices, being physically active, and taking medications can help you reach your targets.

Make Wise Food Choices

Many people find that changing what they eat can make a big difference in their blood glucose, blood pressure, and cholesterol levels. Following are several strategies for making wise food choices:

- Eat less fat, especially saturated fat (found in fatty meats, poultry skin, butter, 2% or whole milk, ice cream, cheese, palm oil, coconut oil, trans-fats, hydrogenated oils, lard, and shortening).
- Choose lean meats and meat substitutes.
- Switch to low-fat or fat-free dairy products.
- Eat at least five servings of fruits and vegetables each day.
- Cut back on foods that are high in cholesterol (such as egg yolks, high-fat meat and poultry, and high-fat dairy products).
- Choose healthier fats that can help lower cholesterol, such as olive oil or canola oil. Nuts also have a healthy type of fat.
- Eat fish two or three times a week, choosing kinds that are high in heart-protective fat (such as albacore tuna, herring, mackerel, rainbow trout, sardines, and wild salmon).
- Cook using low-fat methods (such as baking, roasting, or grilling foods or by using nonstick pans and cooking sprays).
- Eat more foods that are high in fiber (such as oatmeal, oat bran, dried beans and peas such as kidney beans, fruits, and vegetables).
- Eat less salt.
- Cut down on calories and fat.
- Be more physically active; strive for up to 30 minutes of aerobics daily.
- Quit smoking.

Cancer

Cancer develops when cells in the body begin to grow out of control. Normal cells grow, divide, and die. Instead of dying, cancer cells continue to grow and form new abnormal cells. Cancer cells often travel to other body parts, where they grow and replace normal tissue. This process, called metastasis, occurs as the cancer cells get into the bloodstream or lymph vessels. Cancer cells develop because of damage to DNA. DNA is in every cell and directs each cell's activities. When DNA becomes damaged the body is able to repair it. In cancer cells, the damage is not repaired. People can inherit damaged DNA, which accounts for inherited cancers. Many times, DNA becomes damaged by exposure to something in the environment, such as tobacco smoke.[65]

Genetics[66]

- All cancers develop because of genetic alterations of one kind or another. An alteration is a change or mutation in the physical structure of a gene that interferes with the gene's normal functions.

- Some alterations that increase the risk of cancer are present at birth in the genes of all cells in the body, including reproductive cells. These alterations, which are called germline alterations, can be passed from parent to child. This type of alteration is known as an inherited susceptibility and is uncommon as a cause of cancer.

- Most cancers are not due to an inherited susceptibility but result from genetic changes that occur during one's lifetime within the cells of a particular organ.

Skin Cancer

Skin cancer is the most rapidly increasing cancer in the United States, with more than 1 million new cases each year. The most likely reason that skin cancer rates are rising is that people are spending more time outdoors. Ozone layer depletion may also contribute. Using SPF lotion consistently and reapplying when necessary prevents damage to the skin.[67]

Warning Signs
- Any change on the skin.
  - A new spot
  - A spot changes in size, shape, or color
  - A sore that won't heal
  - A mole or dark-colored growth, especially one that looks crusty, or oozes or bleeds.
- Use the ABCDs:
  A = Asymmetry: Does one half of the mole look different than the other half?
  B = Borders: Are the mole's edges ragged or not clearly defined?
  C = Color: Is the mole more than one color?
  D = Diameter: From edge to edge is the mole larger than 6 millimeters?

Risk Factors
- Personal or family history of skin cancer
- Moles
- Natural blonde or red hair color
- Skin sunburns easily

- History of excessive sun exposure, tanning booths, or sunburns
- Occupational exposure to coal tar, pitch, creosote, arsenic compounds, or radium

Prevention

- Limit or avoid the sun from 10 A.M. to 4 P.M. even on cloudy days.
- When outdoors, wear a large hat to shade your face, neck, and ears.
- Wear sunglasses.
- Wear lightweight clothing that covers as much of your body as possible. Don't forget about the tops of your feet!
- Use sunscreen with SPF 15 or higher and reapply sunscreen regularly throughout the day when outdoors. People allergic to PABA should use PABA-free sunscreen.

Breast Cancer

Even though lung cancer and heart disease kill more women each year, surveys show that women view breast cancer as the biggest threat to their health.

Breast cancer occurs when cells in the breast grow out of control. The cells clump together and form a malignant (cancerous) tumor. Most breast tumors are benign, which means they are not cancerous. Benign breast tumors are not life threatening and do not spread outside the breast. Anyone can get breast cancer (including men), but it usually strikes women over age 50. And the risk quickly goes up with age. Women who have a family history of breast cancer have a higher risk.

Symptoms[68]

Breast cancer may not have symptoms in the early stages. But as the cancer grows, the symptoms may include:

- A lump or mass in the breast or the underarm area.
- A change in breast size, shape, or color.
- A discharge from the nipple.
- A change in the feel of the skin covering the breast (the skin could become dimpled, puckered, or scaly).

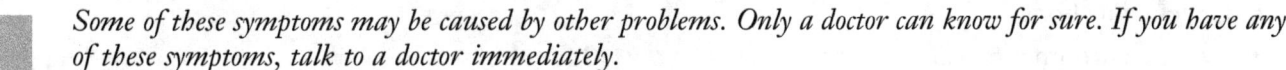

Some of these symptoms may be caused by other problems. Only a doctor can know for sure. If you have any of these symptoms, talk to a doctor immediately.

How Do You Lower Your Risk of Breast Cancer?

- Cut down on the amount of alcohol you drink.
- Maintain a healthy weight.
- Eat more vegetables.
- Perform monthly breast self-examinations.
- Undergo clinical breast exams (every three years for women in their 20s and 30s, every year for women 40+).
- Get a yearly mammogram (for all women starting at age 40, younger if other factors indicate higher risk).

Testicular Cancer

Testicular cancer is the most common cancer in men 20 to 35 years old.

Risk Factors[69]

- Having had an undescended testicle, a condition in which one or both testicles fail to move from the abdomen, where they develop before birth, into the scrotum.
- Having had abnormal development of the testicles.
- Having a personal or family history of testicular cancer.
- Having Klinefelter's syndrome, a genetic disorder in males caused by having an extra X chromosome.
- Being white.

Symptoms

- Enlargement of one testicle
- Dull ache in the lower abdomen or groin
- A painless, lump, or swelling in either testicle
- A change in how the testicle feels
- A sudden buildup of fluid in the scrotum
- Pain or discomfort in a testicle or in the scrotum

Prevention

- Monthly testicular self-exams

How Can You Reduce Cancer Risk?

- Stop smoking!
- Stay out of the sun and sun lamps
- Limit alcohol
- Exercise
- Adhere to a healthy diet
- Watch your weight
- Be sexually cautious
- Check your body
- Avoid environmental carcinogens
- Know your family history

What Is Asthma?[70]

Asthma is a chronic disease that affects your airways, which are the tubes that carry air in and out of your lungs. If you have asthma, the inside walls of your airways are inflamed (swollen). The inflammation makes the airways very sensitive, and they tend to react strongly to things to which you are allergic or find irritating. When the airways react, they get narrower and less air flows through to your lung tissues. This causes symptoms like wheezing (a whistling sound when you breathe), coughing, chest tightness, and trouble breathing.

Asthma cannot be cured, but for most patients it can be controlled so that only minimal and infrequent symptoms occur and an active life can be pursued.

Who Gets Asthma?[71]

In the United States, about 15 million people have asthma. Nearly 5 million of them are children. Asthma is closely linked to allergies. Most, but not all, people with asthma have allergies. Children with a family history of allergies and asthma are more likely to have asthma.

Although asthma affects people of all ages, it often starts in childhood and is more common in children than adults. More boys have asthma than girls, but in adulthood, more women have asthma than men.

Although asthma is a problem among all races, blacks have more asthma attacks and are more likely than whites to be hospitalized for asthma attacks and to die from asthma.

What Are the Symptoms of Asthma?

- **Coughing**—Coughing from asthma is often worse at night or early in the morning, making it hard to sleep.
- **Wheezing**—Wheezing is a whistling or squeaky sound when you breathe.
- **Chest tightness**—This can feel like something is squeezing or sitting on your chest.
- **Shortness of breath**—Some people say they can't catch their breath, or they feel breathless or out of breath. You may feel like you can't get enough air in or out of your lungs.
- **Faster breathing or noisy breathing.**

In addition, people with asthma may have:

- Wheezing when they have a cold or other illness.
- Frequent coughing, especially at night (sometimes this is the only sign of asthma in a child).
- Asthma symptoms brought on by exercise such as running, biking, or other brisk activity, especially during cold weather.
- Coughing or wheezing brought on by prolonged crying or laughing.
- Coughing or wheezing when they are near an allergen or irritant.

If you have asthma, you need to know what things worsen your asthma symptoms. Then do what you can to avoid or limit contact with these things. For example:

- If animal dander is a problem for you, keep your pet out of the house and/or at least out of your bedroom and wash your pet often, or find it a new home.
- Do not smoke or allow smoking in your home.
- If pollen is a problem for you, stay indoors with the air conditioner on when the pollen count is high.
- To control dust mites, wash your sheets, blankets, pillows, and stuffed toys once a week in hot water. You can get special dust-proof covers for your mattress and pillows.
- To prevent colds and flu, wash your hands often and get a flu shot every year. Children with asthma should get flu shots, too.
- If cold air bothers you, wear a scarf over your mouth and nose in the winter.
- If you get asthma when you exercise or do routine physical activities like climbing stairs, work with your doctor to find ways to be active without having asthma symptoms. Physical activity is important.
- If you are allergic to sulfites, avoid foods (like dried fruit) or beverages (like wine) that contain them.

Scientists do not yet know how to prevent the inflammation of the airways that leads to asthma. Scientists are exploring some theories:

- Babies exposed to tobacco smoke are more likely to get asthma. If a mother smokes during pregnancy, her baby may also be more likely to get asthma. Personal smoking may also cause asthma.
- Obesity may be linked to asthma as well as other health problems.
- Environmental contaminants and pollution may cause asthma.

What Is Thyroid Disease?

Your thyroid is a small bowtie- or butterfly-shaped gland, located in your neck, wrapped around the windpipe, behind and below the Adam's Apple area. The thyroid produces several hormones, but two are key: triiodothyronine (T3) and thyroxine (T4). These hormones help oxygen get into cells, and make your thyroid the master gland of metabolism. The thyroid has the only cells in the body capable of absorbing iodine.

Risk Factors for Thyroid Disease

- Women > risk then men
- Age > 50 years
- A personal or family history of thyroid and/or autoimmune disease increases risk
- Being pregnant or within the first year after childbirth
- Current or former smoker
- Radiation exposure
- Recent exposure to iodine via contrast dye or surgical antiseptic
- Recent neck trauma, biopsy, injection or surgery
- High-stress life events

Hypothyroidism

This condition is when the body does not produce enough thyroid hormones to properly regulate metabolism.

Some causes are:

1. Inflammation of the thyroid glands
2. Surgical removal of the entire or parts of the thyroid glands
3. Iodine deficiency
4. Postpartum
5. Hashimoto's is an autoimmune disease in which the thyroid gland is gradually destroyed by a variety of cell and antibody mediated immune processes.

Symptoms:

- Goiter (abnormally enlarged thyroid gland; can result from underproduction or overproduction of hormone or from a deficiency of iodine in the diet)
- Brittle finger nails
- Thin, brittle hair

- Muscle cramps
- Poor muscle tone
- Joint pain
- Weight gain
- Inability to tolerate cold
- Dry, itchy skin
- Decreased production of sweat
- Constipation
- Depression
- Slow speech
- Developing a hoarse voice
- Decreased libido in men

Treatment options:
- Some affected persons are given desiccated thyroid extract produced from the thyroid of an animal such as a pig.

Hyperthyroidism

This is the condition where there is an overabundance of thyroid hormones in the body.

Some causes are:
1. Graves Disease, which results when the immune system attacks the thyroid gland. When this happens, the gland produces too much thyroid hormone to fight the attack.
2. Thyroiditis, an inflammation of the thyroid.

Symptoms:
- Weight loss
- Hyperactivity
- Hair loss
- Depression
- Excessive sweating
- Shortness of breath
- Chest pains
- Heart palpitations
- Moodiness
- Infertility
- Menstrual problems

Treatment options:
Surgical removal (partial or full) of the thyroid gland, the use of medication, or the use of radioiodine. When radioactive iodine is introduced into the body, it kills or severely damages thyroid cells.

Natural Ways to Treat Thyroid Problems

Diet: Eating foods that are high in iodine such as beetroot, radish, potatoes, bananas, nuts and seafood. Limiting the types of foods that increase thyroid hormones, such as RAW cabbage, broccoli, brussels sprouts, sweet potatoes, and lima beans.

Herbs: Some herbs have been found to help control hypothyroidism, such as nettle kelp and bladderwrack, but always consult your doctor before using any herbs.

Exercise: At least 30 minutes of exercise daily is recommended.

Vitamin D: Some amount of vitamin D from the sun is good as it aids in metabolism; or take a supplement.

Health Promotion Planning

Organized healthcare consumers and communities are engaged throughout the country in a wide range of work to improve healthcare access and quality of care, to expand public health, and to reform the healthcare system. Their main focus is on 1) obtaining coverage for the uninsured, 2) increasing access to services at the local level, and 3) improving public health.

Among the most important skills is the ability to plan a community health promotion/disease prevention program. The actions and conditions that protect and improve community or population health can be organized into three areas: health promotion, health protection, and health services.

Health promotion is defined as educational and social efforts designed to help people take greater control of and improve their health. It seeks to activate local organizations and groups or individuals to make changes in lifestyle behaviors, participation in community or political action, and in policies that influence health.

Two areas in which communities employ health promotion strategies are mental and social health, and recreation and fitness. Though both of these health concerns seem to be problems of individuals, a health concern becomes a community or population health concern when many people begin to get sick from the above conditions. For example, eating fast food, although an individual matter, can lead to heart disease or diabetes which becomes a public health problem, where our tax money is going to be spent caring for those sick with lifestyle and preventable diseases.

Action to deal with these concerns begins with a community assessment, which should identify the factors that influence the health of the subpopulations and the needs of these populations.

There are three levels of prevention:

1. **Primary prevention** (measures that forestall the onset of illness)—The goal is to prevent disease from ever occurring. Examples include exercise and meditation classes to enhance nutritional, physical, and mental health.

2. **Secondary prevention** (measures that lead to an early diagnosis and prompt treatment)—The goal is to reduce the severity of disease and prevent disability and death. An example is detecting a bacterial respiratory infection and prescribing antibiotics to combat it.

3. **Tertiary prevention** (measures aimed at rehabilitation following significant pathogenesis)—The goal is to reduce impairment and minimize suffering. Tertiary prevention might take the form of providing rehabilitation services to people involved in an accident.

Health protection and services include the implementing of laws, rules, or policies approved in a community as a result of health promotion or legislation. An example of health protection would be a law to restrict the use of trans fat in food, while an example of health services would be a policy offering free condoms by a local health department. Both of these actions could be the result of health promotion efforts such as a letter writing campaign or members of a community lobbying their board of health.

Community organizing involves bringing people together to combat shared problems and increase their power of decision making. Community organization is intervention whereby individuals, groups, and organizations engage in planned action to influence social problems. It is concerned with the enrichment, development, and/or change of social institutions.

Steps to Organizing a Healthy Community Intervention

Program planning is a process by which an intervention is planned to help meet the needs of a target population.

Assessing the needs of the target population is the first task in creating a health promotion/disease prevention program. You need to know the community you will be working in and the history of the issue you will address. Allow ample time to become familiar with the community, its history, make-up, demographics, geography, and political leadership. One-on-one interviews are an important part of community organizing. The main goal of the one-on-one is to listen and gather information. An organizer needs to meet first with people individually, rather than try to meet everyone in a group.

Step 1 is gathering data.
Step 2 is analyzing the data collected.
Step 3 is prioritizing the identified needs.
Step 4 is validating the need.

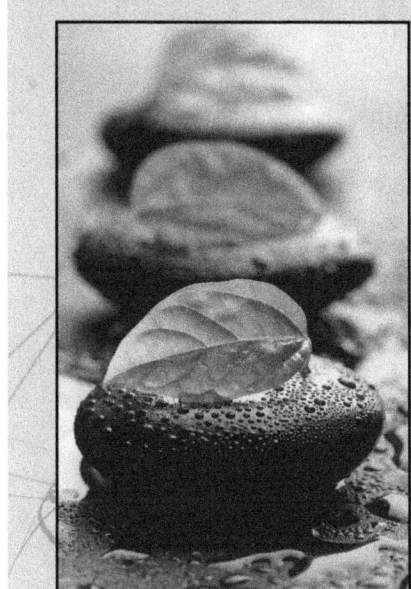

Chapter 3
PSYCHOLOGICAL WELL-BEING

Are You Psychologically Healthy?

1. My sleep has become disturbed—too much, too little, or I wake up constantly.
   ○ Not at all   ○ Somewhat   ○ Quite a lot   ○ Nearly all the time

2. My mood swings from depression to happiness for no reason.
   ○ Not at all   ○ Somewhat   ○ Quite a lot   ○ Nearly all the time

3. I eat more than I should.
   ○ Not at all   ○ Somewhat   ○ Quite a lot   ○ Nearly all the time

4. I enjoy spending time playing a computer or online game more than I enjoy most everything else in my life.
   ○ Not at all   ○ Somewhat   ○ Quite a lot   ○ Nearly all the time

5. People sometimes think that I'm unstable or unreliable.
   ○ Not at all   ○ Somewhat   ○ Quite a lot   ○ Nearly all the time

6. I have poor self-esteem.
   ○ Not at all   ○ Somewhat   ○ Quite a lot   ○ Nearly all the time

7. I often feel that I don't play any useful part in life.
   ○ Not at all   ○ Somewhat   ○ Quite a lot   ○ Nearly all the time

8. I have thought about ending my life.
   ○ Not at all   ○ Somewhat   ○ Quite a lot   ○ Nearly all the time

9. Sometimes I am overwhelmed by distractions or thoughts that I can't seem to control.
   ○ Not at all   ○ Somewhat   ○ Quite a lot   ○ Nearly all the time

10. I often have disturbing dreams or recollections about something that happened in my life.
    ○ Not at all   ○ Somewhat   ○ Quite a lot   ○ Nearly all the time

11. I hate the way I look.
    ○ Not at all   ○ Somewhat   ○ Quite a lot   ○ Nearly all the time

12. I often cry or go into a rage for no reason.
    ○ Not at all   ○ Somewhat   ○ Quite a lot   ○ Nearly all the time

13. My feelings or behaviors are interfering with work, school, friendships, or my relationship.
    ○ Not at all   ○ Somewhat   ○ Quite a lot   ○ Nearly all the time
14. I feel unhappy, sad or worthless.
    ○ Not at all   ○ Somewhat   ○ Quite a lot   ○ Nearly all the time
15. I feel out of control.
    ○ Not at all   ○ Somewhat   ○ Quite a lot   ○ Nearly all the time
16. I often feel empty or that my life has little meaning.
    ○ Not at all   ○ Somewhat   ○ Quite a lot   ○ Nearly all the time
17. Do you ever see or hear things when no one else is around?
    ○ Not at all   ○ Somewhat   ○ Quite a lot   ○ Nearly all the time
18. Do you ever think so fast that when you talk your mouth can't keep up with your thoughts?
    ○ Not at all   ○ Somewhat   ○ Quite a lot   ○ Nearly all the time
19. Do you avoid making friends in case they try and make a fool of you?
    ○ Not at all   ○ Somewhat   ○ Quite a lot   ○ Nearly all the time
20. I am finding it more difficult to cope with things than usual.
    ○ Not at all   ○ Somewhat   ○ Quite a lot   ○ Nearly all the time
21. I am having trouble concentrating at work or school.
    ○ Not at all   ○ Somewhat   ○ Quite a lot   ○ Nearly all the time
22. Based on the above answers, do you think you are psychologically healthy? Why or why not?

_____

_____

_____

_____

_____

_____

23. What psychological areas need improvement in your life?

_____

_____

_____

_____

_____

_____

Definition of Psychological Health

If you aren't sick or do not have any disease, it doesn't mean you are healthy. According to the World Health Organization (WHO), health is a state of complete physical, mental, and social well-being and not merely the absence of disease or infirmity.

So are you psychologically feeling well right now?

_____

_____

_____

_____

_____

Dimensions of Psychological Health

- Mental
- Emotional
- Spiritual
- Cultural

How would you describe your level of self-esteem?

_____

_____

_____

_____

_____

Self-Esteem

- Belief and pride in ourselves
- Ability to maintain, and often regain, a positive view of one's self, no matter what
- External factors versus internal factors
- Allows us to try things we've failed at and take on new challenges

Boosting Self-Esteem

- Receive/provide unconditional love
- Set realistic expectations
- Provide positive affirmations
- Give compliments and encouragement

Definition of Stress

To your body, *stress* is synonymous with change. Stress is the emotional and physical symptoms that individuals experience as the result of change. Stress may be considered as any physical, chemical, or emotional factor that causes bodily or mental tension and that may be a factor in disease causation. The majority of visits to physicians are because of stress-related complaints.

Stress can be positive or negative (eustress vs. distress). A mild degree of stress and tension can sometimes be beneficial.

Symptoms of Stress

- Rapid heart rate
- Headaches, backaches
- Muscular aches
- Sweating
- Tics
- Insomnia
- Fatigue
- High blood pressure
- Impotence and other sexual problems
- Dizziness
- Depression, anxiety
- Irritation, anger, hostility
- Fear, panic attacks
- Poor concentration
- More infections, illnesses

What Happens to Our Bodies Under Stress?

- *Brain*—headaches, anxiety, depression, insomnia, memory loss
- *Digestive system*—slows down, mouth ulcers or cold sores, upset stomach
- *Heart*—Increased heart rate, increased blood pressure
- *Skin*—breakouts, rashes, itching, eczema

- *Muscle*—tension, tics
- *Reproductive system*—menstrual disorders, infertility in females; impotence, premature ejaculation in males.

Stress and the Immune System

- Powerful chemicals triggered by stress suppress the immune system, making the body more susceptible to illness.
- Stress interferes with the body's ability to heal.
- Increased adrenaline production causes the body to increase metabolism of proteins, fats, and carbohydrates to quickly produce energy for the body to use.
- The pituitary gland increases production of andrenocorticotropic hormone (ACTH), which in turn stimulates the release of cortisone and cortisol hormones. These hormonal releases may inhibit the functioning of disease-fighting white blood cells and suppress the immune system's response.

Health Disorders Associated with Chronic Stress

- Coronary heart disease
- Hypertension
- Diabetes
- Progression of breast cancer
- Ulcers
- Eating disorders
- Asthma
- Depression
- Migraines
- Sleep disorders
- Chronic fatigue
- Physical aches, pains

Selye's Model—General Adaptation Syndrome

Stressor = Alarm + Resistance + Exhaustion

Our bodies try to keep in balance (homeostasis), but stress may upset that balance. Hans Selye explained stress through GAS (general adaptation syndrome), a way that the body tries to keep in balance.

A stressor is anything that affects you emotionally or physically.

Examples of Stressors

- School
- Work
- Parents
- Relationships

- Road rage
- Illness and disability
- Death of a loved one
- Discrimination
- Violence
- War
- Other

The *alarm stage* is when your body is preparing to defend itself against the stressor. Your body will go into "fight or flight" response by releasing hormones such as adrenaline and insulin to allow you to flee or attack. Heart rate and blood pressure will be elevated. In ancient times, a stressor such as being chased by a tiger would be beneficial by allowing the release of adrenaline hormones to allow for running away or killing the tiger.

The *resistance stage* allows arousal to be elevated while the body is trying to defend itself against the stressor.

The *exhaustion stage* occurs when resources are limited or depleted and the ability to resist the stressor is impaired. This stage leads to increased vulnerability of health problems and an impaired immune system.

Personality Types and Stress

- *Type A*—aggressive, hard-driven, impatient; high levels of distress. Prone to stress-related diseases such as ulcers, heart disease, hypertension, and certain cancers.
- *Type B*—easygoing, laid-back, patient; low levels of distress.
- *Type C*—passive, apologetic, overly sensitive; moderate levels of distress. Prone to stress-related mental disorders.
- *Type D*—tendency toward negativity; may experience a lot of stress, anger, worry, hostility, tension, and other negative and distressing emotions. Prone to depression, heart disease, hypertension.

Stress May Trigger Anger

Researchers believe that prolonged stress and anger result in the breakdown of the cardiovascular system. It can also increase your risk for developing mental health concerns such as:

- Depression
- Eating disorders
- Drug, alcohol, or other addictions
- Suicidal thoughts
- Relationship problems

You might be holding in anger and not even be aware of it. Do you find yourself flying off the handle on a regular basis or having road rage or screaming or exploding at the littlest things that aggravate you? Anger is caused by an irrational perception of reality and a low frustration point. Angry people almost never admit responsibility—they blame something or someone else for their anger. When you are in the angry "rage"—it's hard to think clearly because your emotions take control of your actions. The fight or flight response takes over and increases blood pressure and heart rate and releases adrenaline into your bloodstream, which tells your body to either defend yourself or attack someone/something.

How to Control Your Anger

- Breathe deeply, from your diaphragm.
- Slowly repeat a calming word or phrase such as "relax" or "calm."
- Use imagery; visualize a relaxing experience.
- Exercise or yoga to release the adrenaline.
- Take a "time out"—leave the scene and cool off.
- Talk with a psychologist to improve your problem-solving skills.

How to Deal With an Angry Person

1. Become an impartial observer—act as if you were watching someone else.
2. Stay calm—do not add fuel to the fire.
3. Refuse to engage.
4. Defuse them by ignoring them, looking away, or starting another conversation with a totally different topic, or find something you can agree with or praise them.
5. Walk away if the person is getting out of control.
6. Practice your deep breathing.

How to Change Your Personality to Become More Stress-Resilient

- Build greater social support networks.
- Participate in and contribute to your community in productive ways.
- Set clear boundaries and expectations for yourself.
- Develop decision-making skills.
- Practice effective communication techniques.
- Learn conflict management techniques.
- Do not try to control the outcome of every situation.

Hardiness—health authorities have now identified the concept of hardiness as a characteristic that has helped people negate self-imposed stress.

One researcher in the stress hardiness field is Susan Kobasa, PhD, the clinical psychologist at City University, New York. In the late 1970s she carried out a study on a group of executives who were under a lot of stress while their company, the Bell Telephone Company, was undergoing radical restructuring. On completion of the study, when the data was analyzed, she found that certain personality traits protected some of the executives and managers from the health ravages of stress.

These stress-hardy personality traits included:

1. Commitment—having a purpose to life and involvement in family, work, community, social friends, religious faith, ourselves, etc., giving us meaning to our lives.
2. Control—studies have shown that how much control we perceive we have over any stressor will influence how difficult the stressor will be for us to cope with.
3. Challenge—how we perceive the events that occur in our lives; seeing our difficulties as a challenge rather than as a threat, and accepting that the only thing in life that is constant, is change.

Definitions

Hormone: A chemical substance released into the body by the endocrine glands such as the thyroid, adrenal, or ovaries. The substance travels through the bloodstream and sets in motion various body functions. For example, prolactin, produced in the pituitary gland, begins and sustains the production of breastmilk after childbirth.

Neurotransmitters: Specialized chemical messengers (e.g., acetylcholine, dopamine, norepinephrine, serotonin) that send messages from one nerve cell to another. Most neurotransmitters play different roles throughout the body, many of which are not yet known.

Neurotransmitters are molecules that regulate brain function. They are chemicals that relay messages from nerve to nerve both within the brain and outside the brain. They also relay messages from nerve to muscle, lungs, and intestinal tracts. They can accentuate *emotion, thought processes, joy, elation,* and also *fear, anxiety, insomnia,* and the terrible urge to *overindulge* in food, alcohol, drugs, and so on. In short, neurotransmitters are used all over the body to transmit information and signals. They are manufactured and used by neurons (nerve cells) and are released into the synaptic clefts between the neurons.

Currently, over 50 neurotransmitters have been identified, and it is estimated that around 100 neurotransmitters exist in the biological systems.

Stress Hormones/Neurotransmitters

Epinephrine, also known as **adrenaline**, the major stress neurotransmitter, is related to blood pressure and heart rate. Adrenaline prepares the body for "fright, fight, or flight" responses and has many effects, including:

- Action of heart increased
- Rate and depth of breathing increased
- Metabolic rate increased
- Force of muscular contraction improves
- Onset of muscular fatigue delayed

Norepinephrine, also known as **noradrenaline**, is a second stress neurotransmitter. High levels of this hormone are seen in states of anxiety and insomnia. It is released in response to perceived threat. The effects of the hormone noradrenaline are similar to the effects of adrenaline, the other hormone secreted by the adrenal medulla.

The actions of noradrenaline include:

- Constriction of small blood vessels leading to increase in blood pressure
- Increased blood flow through the coronary arteries and slowing of heart rate
- Increase in rate and depth of breathing

Increased amounts of both adrenaline and noradrenaline are secreted when the body is under stress.

Cortisol is secreted in times of stress. Cortisol stimulates fat and carbohydrate metabolism for fast energy, and stimulates insulin release and maintenance of blood sugar levels. The end result of these actions is *an increase in appetite*, especially cravings for sugared foods. Cortisol increases abdominal obesity. Cortisol secretion is highest in people who sleep less than six hours per night.

Major "Happy" Neurotransmitters

- **Endorphins** (opioids): Provides mood-elevating, enhancing, and euphoric effects. The more endorphins present, the happier you are! Endorphins are like natural painkillers—your body's natural heroin.
- **Dopamine**: Runs your body's pleasure center. Creates feelings of bliss and pleasure, euphoria, and focus. Also leads to appetite control and controlled motor movements. Modulates the effect of the excitatory hormones, and is necessary for states of relaxation and mental alertness.
- **Serotonin**: Manufactured from tryptophan. It is found all over the body and is necessary to modulate the levels of the stress hormones. Promotes and improves sleep, improves self-esteem, relieves depression, diminishes craving, and prevents agitated depression and worrying. Converts to melatonin and then back to serotonin. Regulates your body clock. First to fail under stress.
- **Melatonin**: "Rest and recuperation" and "antiaging" hormone. Regulates body clock.
- **Acetylcholine**: Affects alertness, memory, and sexual performance; stimulates appetite control, and release of growth hormone.
- **Phenylethylamine** (PEA): Provides feelings of bliss, feelings of infatuation (high levels are found in chocolate).
- **Oxytocin**: Stimulated by dopamine. Promotes sexual arousal, feelings of emotional attachment, and desire to cuddle.
- **GABA** (*gamma amino butyric acid*): Found throughout central nervous system, produces antistress, antianxiety, antipanic, and antipain effects. Allows individual to feel calm, maintain control, and focus.

Neurotransmitters control

- Nicotine craving
- Premenstrual syndrome (PMS)
- Irritable bowel
- Caffeine craving
- ADHD
- Anorexia and bulimia
- Migraine headache
- Panic attacks
- Alcohol craving
- Leg cramps
- Constipation
- Carbohydrate cravings
- OCD
- Aggression
- Impulsivity

How Stress Affects Neurotransmitters

The brain uses feel-good transmitters called **endorphins** when managing daily stress. When the brain requires larger amounts of endorphins to handle increased stress, the ratio of many of the other transmitters, one to another, becomes upset, creating a chemical imbalance. We begin to feel stress more acutely—a sense of urgency and anxiety creates even more stress. As long as the brain has a balanced amount of happy and sad messengers, everything runs smoothly and we are in homeostasis.

It is imperative that all of the major neurotransmitters be present daily and in sufficient amounts in order for the brain to be chemically balanced. When insufficient amounts of one or more of these neurotransmitters exists, it upsets the ratio and symptoms are experienced.

Depleted supplies of feel-good transmitters means it will be impossible for you to feel happy, upbeat, motivated, or on track. You will feel just the opposite: a decrease in energy and interest, feelings of worthlessness, and a pervasive sense of helplessness to control the course of your life.

Certain transmitters, when depleted, may cause you to be easily agitated or angered, experience mild to severe anxiety, and have sleep problems. You may feel more psychological and physical pain. These are all possible symptoms of neurotransmitter deficiencies.

Main Causes of Neurotransmitter Deficiencies

- *Genetics*: A person's genetic makeup is responsible for low, high, or balanced levels of transmitters from birth.

- *Stress*: Stress depletes neurotransmitters! Any type of stress (lack of sleep, everyday mental and emotional battles, or poor health) will deplete feel-good transmitters. This results in a reduction of transmitters needed for sleep, as well as a reduction in pain-blocking transmitters.

- *Diet*: The specific amino acids that our brains manufacture transmitters from are frequently not supplied by our modern diet or in the way our brain best utilizes them. Nutrient-depleted soils, fruits and vegetables not allowed to fully ripen on the vine, and overprocessing of foods have all combined over the last century to rob our diets of many life-giving nutrients. Experts in the field of brain nutrition all agree that it is very difficult to get the necessary supply of the specific amino acids from our American diet that our brain needs to create enough of the neurotransmitters that keep us feeling balanced and happy.

How to Treat Neurotransmitter Imbalance

If we treat a neurotransmitter imbalance with pharmaceutical medication (i.e., the serotonin reuptake inhibitors like Prozac, Celexa, Paxil, and Zoloft), we tend to impose an artificial and imbalanced level of a specific neurotransmitter.

These drugs will increase the amount of serotonin at the synaptic cleft, causing the body to *think* that serotonin levels are higher. Most people will feel better temporarily. When serotonin stores fall below a certain level, the medication "stops working" and a different medication must be used. However, they do *not increase the total body stores of serotonin*, and therefore are not the best permanent solution.

Alternatives to Medication

1. Increase dietary intake of tryptophan. American diets tend to be high in carbohydrate and low in protein. Foods high in tryptophan are mostly high-protein foods:
   - Cottage cheese—450 mg per cup
   - Fish and other seafood—800–1,300 mg per pound
   - Meats—1,000–1,300 mg per pound

- Poultry—600–1,200 mg per pound
- Peanuts, roasted with skin—800 mg per cup
- Sesame seeds—700 mg per cup
- Dry, whole lentils—450 mg per cup

2. Increase amount of exercise. Exercise leads to more efficient use of insulin, thus reducing insulin resistance and decreasing the amount of food that is stored as fat. When the cells process nutrients better, they make neurotransmitters better. Exercise releases endorphins, which are natural mood elevators.

3. Reduce our intake of caffeine. Caffeine makes the body think is it under stress, which raises the cortisol level, raises the insulin level, and causes carbohydrates to be deposited as fat.

Functions of Endorphins

Endorphins, chemicals produced in the brain in response to a variety of stimuli, may be nature's cure for high levels of stress.

Endorphins are among the brain chemicals known as neurotransmitters, which, as noted, function in the transmission of signals within the nervous system. At least 20 types of endorphins have been demonstrated in humans, and they may be located in the pituitary gland, other parts of the brain, or distributed throughout the nervous system.

Stress and pain are the two most common factors leading to the release of endorphins. Endorphins interact with the opiate receptors in the brain to reduce our perception of pain, having a similar action to drugs such as morphine and codeine. Unlike drugs, however, activation of the opiate receptors by the body's endorphins does not lead to addiction or dependence.

Results of Endorphin Secretion

- Decreased feelings of pain
- Feelings of euphoria
- Modulation of appetite
- Release of sex hormones
- Enhancement of the immune response

Stress and Digestion

Stress contributes to ulcers and ailing digestion.

- Good nutrition can help.
- Complex carbohydrates increase levels of serotonin.
- Stay hydrated with water to compensate for fluid lost during sweating under stress and stress-induced dry mouth.
- Eat frequent, small meals to maintain normal blood sugar, prevent fatigue and irritability, and prevent slow metabolism.
- Avoid overeating, which can increase stress.
- Limit consumption of sugar, caffeine, nicotine, and alcohol.

Vitamin and Mineral Deficiencies

Chronic stress can deplete several vitamins necessary for energy metabolism, as well as those necessary for the stress response itself. The stress response activates several hormones responsible for mobilizing and metabolizing fats and carbohydrates for energy production. The breakdown of fats and carbohydrates requires vitamins, specifically the B vitamins and vitamin C. An inadequate supply of these may affect mental alertness, promote depression, and lead to insomnia. Stress is also associated with the depletion of calcium and the inability of bones to absorb it properly.

"Pick-Me-Ups" and Stress

When people are stressed, they use *pick-me-ups* or *put-me-downs* to combat the stressor. Several substances tend to either mimic or induce the stress response, or decrease the efficiency of the body's metabolic pathways, thus setting the stage for more pronounced physiological reactions to stress. The biggest mistake people make in handling stress is using pick-me-ups to boost happy messengers, which has the effect of riding a wild roller coaster.

Sugar: Excess sugar tends to deplete vitamin stores, especially the B vitamins that are crucial for optimal function of the central nervous system. Depletion of B vitamins may result in fatigue, anxiety, and irritability. In addition, excess simple sugars can cause major fluctuations in blood glucose levels, resulting in pronounced fatigue, headaches, and irritability.

Simple Sugars

- Glucose (honey)
- Lactose (milk)
- Fructose (fruit)
- Sucrose (cane)

Fats: You've likely heard all the bad news about how fat creates artery-clogging cholesterol and weight gain. But a high-fat diet also leaves you feeling lethargic and just not feeling as well as you would on a diet high in complex carbohydrates.

Caffeine: Caffeine stimulates the release of several stress hormones, resulting in a state of hyper- alertness, and makes a person more likely to interpret events as stressful.

Alcohol: Increases short-term energy, but then blood sugar dips. Diminishes pain, but can lead to aggression and depression.

Salt: High sodium acts to increase water retention, and as water volume increases, blood pressure increases. Habitual high sodium intake may contribute to hypertension.

Tobacco: Powerful toxin; destroys trachea, bronchi, and lung function. Damages arteries, causing insufficient blood supply to the brain, heart, and organs. Carcinogenic. Increases dopamine but levels fall shortly, requiring more nicotine.

Drugs: Increases release of dopamine (pleasure center), shutting off brain's natural supply.

Your own adrenaline: Allows body to prepare for fight or flight. For example, a workaholic who is over-stressed ➤ works longer hours ➤ feeds off his own adrenaline.

Put-Me-Downs

 "Doctor, can you give me something to calm me down?"

Medications that temporarily force the body into sleeping, producing a tranquilizing effect, are referred to as **put-me-downs**. These medications produce addiction and severe withdrawal symptoms.

- Valium, Xanax, Ativan
- Barbiturates

Stress Interventions

1. Do a minimum of 30 minutes of aerobic exercise daily, or take a walk.
2. Make your body clock regular.
3. Eat five small, balanced meals per day.
4. Avoid caffeine, drugs, and tobacco.
5. Reduce intake of refined sugars and alcohol.
6. Sleep about eight hours nightly.
7. Spend time each day with relaxation techniques—imagery, daydreaming, prayer, or meditation.
8. Take a warm bath or shower.
9. Listen to music; watch a comedy.
10. Postpone making changes in your life.
11. Hug someone, hold hands, or stroke a pet.
12. Pray.

Techniques to Handle Stress

1. *Deep breathing*: Inhale through your nose slowly, counting silently to five, and then exhale through your mouth slowly, counting silently to five.
2. *Positive affirmations*: Talk in a positive manner to yourself; turn your negative comments into positive ones: *"I will pass the test."*
3. *Stretching*: Stretch the area where tension has built up, holding for 30 seconds; relax and repeat three to five times.
4. *Progressive muscle relaxation*: Tense a muscle and hold it for a silent, slow count of 5–10 seconds, then release the muscle for a silent, slow count 5–10 seconds.
5. *Visualization*: Find a quiet space, get comfortable, close your eyes, and try to imagine yourself in a calm, enjoyable, relaxing setting. Think about the details of your tranquil setting. Who is with you? How is the weather? What does it smell like?
6. *Meditation*: Find a quiet space, get comfortable, close your eyes, and begin breathing deeply. Focus on one image or thought. Try this for 5–10 minutes every day.
7. *Yoga*: Used since ancient times to invigorate the body and calm the mind.
8. *Massage*: Research indicates that human touch is vital for well-being.
9. *Pets*: Animals decrease stress levels through touch, companionship.
10. *Talk to someone*: A friend, parent, teacher, or a college counselor.

Dr. Abraham Maslow, father of humanistic psychology, has shed light on various characteristics prevalent in a healthy and psychologically happy person. Dr. Maslow stressed that you need to meet and satisfy lower and basic needs like safety, health, belonging, love, and status before proceeding to higher values. Once people meet these basic needs, they have opportunities for self-exploration and expression that can lead them to reach their fullest human potential. According to Maslow, a self-actualized person is realistic, self-accepting, self-motivated, creative, and capable of intimacy. Those who reach this level achieve a sense of happiness, or well-being, that comes from finding purpose and meaning in life.

Maslow has set up a hierarchy of five levels of basic needs. Beyond these needs, higher levels of needs exist. These include needs for understanding, esthetic appreciation and purely spiritual needs. In the levels of the five basic needs, the person does not feel the second need until the demands of the first have been satisfied, nor the third until the second has been satisfied, and so on. Maslow's model indicates that fundamental, lower-order needs like safety and physiological requirements have to be satisfied in order to pursue higher-level motivators along the lines of self-fulfillment. As depicted in the following hierarchical diagram, sometimes called "Maslow's Needs Pyramid" or "Maslow's Needs Triangle," after a need is satisfied it stops acting as a motivator and the next need one rank higher starts to motivate.

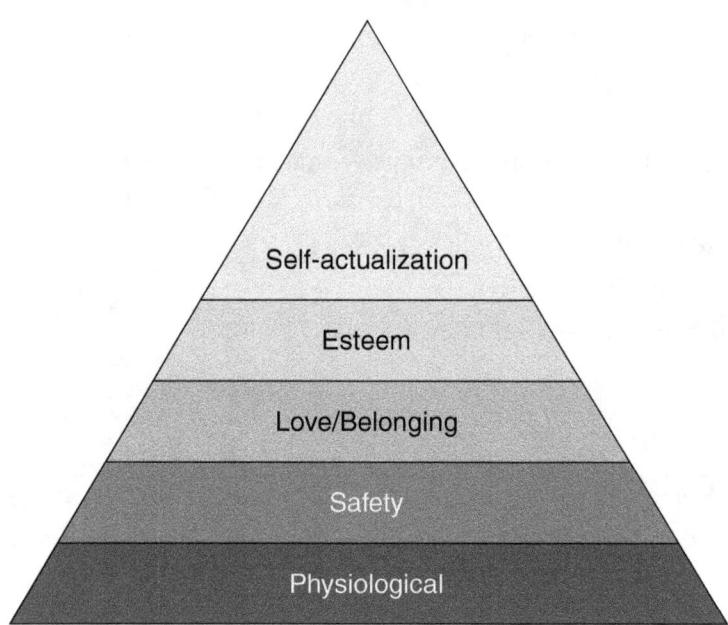

Need for Self-Actualization

Maslow describes self-actualization as a person's need to be and do that which the person was "born to do. A musician must make music, an artist must paint, and a poet must write." These needs make themselves felt in signs of restlessness. The person feels on edge, tense, lacking something; in short—restless.

Need for Esteem

These involve needs for both self-esteem and for the esteem a person gets from others. Humans have a need for a stable, firmly based, high level of self-respect, and respect from others. When these needs are satisfied, the person feels self-confident and valuable as a person in the world. When these needs are frustrated, the person feels inferior, weak, helpless and worthless.

Need for Love, Affection, and Belonging

Maslow states that people seek to overcome feelings of loneliness and alienation. This involves both giving and receiving love, affection, and the sense of belonging.

Safety Need

When all physiological needs are satisfied and are no longer controlling thoughts and behaviors, the need for security can become active.

Physiological Needs

These are biological needs. They consist of needs for oxygen, food, water, and a relatively constant body temperature. They are the strongest needs because if a person were deprived of all needs, the physiological ones would come first in the person's search for satisfaction.

Maslow states that educators should respond to the potential an individual has for growing into a self-actualizing person of his/her own kind. Ten points are:

1. We should teach people to be *authentic,* to be aware of their inner selves and to hear their inner-feeling voices.

2. We should teach people to *transcend their cultural conditioning* and become world citizens.

3. We should help people *discover their vocation in life,* their calling, fate or destiny. This is especially focused on finding the right career and the right mate.

4. We should teach people that *life is precious,* that there is joy to be experienced in life, and if people are open to seeing the good and joyous in all kinds of situations, it makes life worth living.

5. We must *accept the person* as he or she is and help the person learn their inner nature. From real knowledge of aptitudes and limitations we can know what to build upon, what potentials are really there.

6. We must see that the person's *basic needs are satisfied.* This includes safety, belongingness, and esteem needs.

7. We should *refreshen consciousness,* teaching the person to appreciate beauty and the other good things in nature and in living.

8. We should teach people that *controls are good,* and complete abandon is bad. It takes control to improve the quality of life in all areas.

9. We should teach people to transcend the trifling problems and *grapple with the serious problems in life.* These include the problems of injustice, of pain, suffering, and death.

10. We must teach people to be *good choosers.* They must be given practice in making good choices.

Happiness

- A sense of well-being, a feeling that life as a whole is going well
- "Feel-good" versus "value-based"

I feel happy when:

_____

_____

_____

_____

_____

_____

Factors Affecting Happiness

- Genetics
- Relationships
- Gender and race
- Life events
- Education and intelligence
- Age, health, and wealth

Best Predictors of Happiness

- High self-esteem
- Optimism
- Extroversion
- Supportive relationships
- Sense of being in control

Bottom line: Feeling good does not necessarily depend on money, success, recognition, or status. Instead:

- Accept yourself.
- Respect yourself.
- Trust yourself.
- Love yourself.

What is the difference between everyday stressors and mental disorders?

According to the *Diagnostic and Statistical Manual of Mental Disorders (DSM-IV-TR)*, a mental disorder is a pattern of behavior in an individual that is associated with distress or disability or with significantly increased risk of suffering, death, pain, or loss of freedom. A mental disorder differs from everyday stressors or problems because a mental disorder can be diagnosed from a set of symptoms. Worries, fears, anxieties are common, especially during the college years. Most people gradually learn how to deal with life's problems through positive behavior change.

Mental Disorders

Mental disorders include diagnosable mental, behavioral, or emotional disorders that interfere with one or more major activities. One of every two Americans who need mental health treatment do not receive it, and the rate is even lower—and the quality of care poorer—for ethnic and racial minorities.

Panic Attacks

Panic disorder is characterized by unexpected and repeated episodes of intense fear accompanied by physical symptoms that may include chest pain, heart palpitations, shortness of breath, dizziness, or abdominal distress. These sensations often mimic symptoms of a heart attack.

Occurrence

- In a given year 1.7 percent of the U.S. population (2.4 million Americans) experiences panic disorder.
- Women are twice as likely as men to develop panic disorder.
- Panic disorder typically strikes in young adulthood. Roughly half of all people who have panic disorder develop the condition before age 24.[12]

Causes

- Heredity
- Biological
- Catastrophic thinking

Treatment

- Cognitive behavioral therapy: breathing, counting backwards, distraction
- Medication

Anxiety Disorder

Generalized anxiety disorder (GAD) is characterized by six months or more of chronic, exaggerated worry and tension that is unfounded or much more severe than the normal anxiety most people experience. People with this disorder usually expect the worst; they worry excessively about money, health, family, or work, even when there are no signs of trouble. They are unable to relax and often suffer from insomnia. Many people with GAD also have physical symptoms, such as fatigue, trembling, muscle tension, headaches, irritability, or hot flashes.

Occurrence

- About 2.8 percent of the U.S. population (4 million Americans) has GAD during a year's time.
- GAD most often strikes people in childhood or adolescence, but can begin in adulthood, too.
- GAD affects women more often than men.

Causes

- Stress
- Biological

Treatment

- Cognitive behavioral therapy
- Medication
- National Institute of Mental Health (NIMH) Anxiety Information Line: 1-888-8ANXIETY (826-9438)
- NIMH Panic Information Line: 1-888-64PANIC (647-2642)

Obsessive-Compulsive Disorder (OCD)

Individuals with OCD suffer intensely from recurrent, unwanted thoughts (obsessions) or rituals (compulsions) that they feel they cannot control. Rituals such as handwashing, counting, checking, or cleaning are often performed in hopes of preventing obsessive thoughts or making them go away. Performing these rituals, however, provides only temporary relief, and not performing them markedly increases anxiety. Left untreated, obsessions and the need to perform rituals can take over a person's life. OCD is often a chronic, relapsing illness.

Occurrence

- About 2.3 percent of the U.S. population (3.3 million Americans) has OCD in a given year.
- OCD affects men and women equally.

- OCD typically begins during adolescence or early childhood; at least one-third of the cases of adult OCD began in childhood.
- OCD cost the United States $8.4 billion in 1990 in social and economic losses, nearly 6 percent of the total mental health bill of $148 billion.

Causes

- Biological

Treatment

- Behavioral therapy
- Medications

Depression

Depression is the most common mental ailment in the world. Depression causes people to lose pleasure from daily life, can complicate other medical conditions, and can even be serious enough to lead to suicide. Depression is characterized as a sadness that does not end.

Symptoms

- Persistent sad, anxious or "empty" mood
- Sleeping too much or too little; middle of the night or early morning waking
- Reduced appetite and weight loss, or increased appetite and weight gain
- Loss of pleasure and interest in activities once enjoyed, including sex
- Restlessness, irritability
- Persistent physical symptoms that do not respond to treatment (such as chronic pain or digestive disorders)
- Difficulty concentrating, remembering, or making decisions
- Fatigue or loss of energy, feeling guilty, hopeless, or worthless
- Thoughts of suicide or death

> *If you have five or more of these symptoms for two weeks or more, you could have clinical depression and should see your doctor or a qualified mental health professional for help.*

Occurrence

- Clinical depression is one of the most common mental illnesses, affecting more than 19 million Americans each year.
- Depression can affect anyone, at any age, and people of any race or ethnic group.
- Teens born in the 1980s are more likely to develop depression than those who were born in the 1970s, whose rate of depression is higher than those born in the 1960s.[19]

Causes

- *Biological*—People with depression typically have too little or too much of certain brain chemicals, called *neurotransmitters*. Changes in these brain chemicals may cause or contribute to clinical depression.
- *Cognitive*—People with negative thinking patterns and low self-esteem are more likely to develop clinical depression.

- *Gender*—Women experience clinical depression at a rate that is nearly twice that of men. Though the reasons for this are still unclear, they may include the hormonal changes women go through during menstruation, pregnancy, childbirth, and menopause. Other reasons may include the stress caused by the multiple responsibilities that women have.
- *Co-occurrence*—Clinical depression is more likely to occur along with certain illnesses, such as heart disease, cancer, Parkinson's disease, diabetes, Alzheimer's disease, and hormonal disorders.
- *Medications*—Side effects of some medications can bring about depression.
- *Genetic*—A family history of clinical depression increases the risk for developing the illness.
- *Situational*—Difficult life events, including divorce, financial problems or the death of a loved one, can contribute to clinical depression.

Treatment

- Psychotherapy
- Medication

Why do you think so many young people are depressed?

_____

_____

_____

_____

_____

Tips for Dealing with Depression for College Students

- Carefully plan your day.
- Get enough sleep.
- Exercise.
- Participate in extracurricular activities.
- Seek support from other people.
- Try relaxation methods.
- Take time for yourself every day.
- Seek treatment, such as through a college counseling center.

Bipolar Disorder

Bipolar disorder, also known as manic depression, is an illness involving one or more episodes of serious mania and depression. The illness causes a person's mood to swing from excessively "high" and/or irritable to sad and hopeless, with periods of a normal mood in between. More than two million Americans suffer from bipolar disorder.

Symptoms

- Excessive energy, activity, restlessness, racing thoughts, and rapid talking
- Denial that anything is wrong
- Extreme "high" or euphoric feelings
- Easily irritated or distracted
- Decreased need for sleep
- Unrealistic beliefs in one's ability and powers
- Uncharacteristically poor judgment
- Sustained period of behavior that is different from usual
- Unusual sexual drive
- Abuse of drugs, particularly cocaine, alcohol, or sleeping medications
- Provocative, intrusive, or aggressive behavior

Occurrence

- Typically begins in adolescence or early adulthood and continues throughout life

Causes

- Genetic
- Biochemical

Treatment

- Professional help
- Medication
- Support from family, friends, and peers

Suicide

Suicide is not a psychiatric disorder, but it is the consequence of psychological problems.

Occurrence

- Approximately 30,000 Americans commit suicide annually; an additional 752,000 Americans attempt suicide annually; there may be 4.5 million suicide survivors in the United States.
- Women attempt more suicides, but men are more successful.
- Suicide is the third leading cause of death in young adults.

Warning Signs

- Verbal threats
- Expressions of hopelessness and helplessness
- Previous suicide attempts
- Daring or risk-taking behavior
- Personality changes
- Depression
- Giving away possessions
- Lack of interest in future plans

Factors That Protect Against Suicide

- Feeling connected to family and friends
- Emotional well-being
- Avoiding drugs and alcohol

What to do if you think someone is suicidal

- Trust your instincts that the person may be in trouble.
- Talk with the person about your concerns. Communication needs to include *listening*.
- Ask direct questions without being judgmental. Determine if the person has a specific plan to carry out the suicide. The more detailed the plan, the greater the risk.
- Get professional help, even if the person resists.
- Contact the hotline at 1-800-SUICIDE (1-800-784-2433) or www.hopeline.com. This will connect you with a crisis center in your area.
- Do not leave the person alone.
- Do not swear to secrecy.
- Do not act shocked or judgmental.
- Do not counsel the person yourself.

Attention Deficit/Hyperactivity Disorder (ADHD)

Signs and Symptoms

- Impulsiveness
- Inattention
- Hyperactivity

Occurrence

- Three times as many boys as girls are affected by ADHD.

Causes

- Genetic
- Biological
- Differences within the brain
- Prenatal use of tobacco, alcohol, or cocaine
- Delivery complications
- Postnatal illnesses

Treatment

- Behavioral therapy
- Medication

Schizophrenia

Someone with schizophrenia may have difficulty distinguishing between what is real and what is imaginary, may be unresponsive or withdrawn, and may have difficulty expressing normal emotions in social situations.

Signs and Symptoms

- Delusions—false ideas; individuals may believe that someone is spying on them, or that they are someone famous.
- Hallucinations—seeing, feeling, tasting, hearing, or smelling something that doesn't really exist. The most common experience is hearing imaginary voices that give commands or comments to the individual.
- Disordered thinking and speech—moving quickly from one topic to another, in a nonsensical fashion. Individuals may make up their own words or sounds.
- Social withdrawal
- Extreme apathy
- Lack of drive or initiative
- Emotional unresponsiveness[25]

Occurrence

- Mean age for development is 21.4 in men and 26.8 in women.

Causes

- Genetics (heredity)
- Biology (imbalance in the brain's chemistry)
- Viral infections and immune disorders

Treatment

- No cure exists
- Antipsychotic medication
- Psychiatric counseling
- Housing programs
- Case management

Seasonal Affective Disorder (SAD)

Some people suffer from symptoms of depression during the winter months, with symptoms subsiding during the spring and summer months. As seasons change, there is a shift in our "biological internal clocks" or circadian rhythm, due partly to these changes in sunlight patterns. This can cause our biological clocks to be out of step with our daily schedules. The most difficult months for SAD sufferers are January and February, and younger persons and women are at higher risk.

Signs and Symptoms

- Regularly occurring symptoms of depression (excessive eating and sleeping, weight gain) during the fall or winter months.
- Full remission from depression in the spring and summer months.
- Symptoms have occurred in the past two years, with no nonseasonal depression episodes.
- Seasonal episodes substantially outnumber nonseasonal depression episodes.
- A craving for sugary and/or starchy foods.

Causes

Melatonin, a sleep-related hormone secreted by the pineal gland in the brain, has been linked to SAD. This hormone, which may cause symptoms of depression, is produced at increased levels in the dark. Therefore, when the days are shorter and darker the production of this hormone increases.

Treatment

- Phototherapy or bright light therapy
- One hour's walk in winter sunlight
- Antidepressant drugs

Social Anxiety

Social Anxiety is characterized by overwhelming anxiety and excessive self-consciousness in everyday social situations.

Signs and Symptoms

- Persistent, intense, and chronic fear of being watched and judged by others
- Feeling embarrassment or humiliation over own actions
- Fear interferes with work or school or other ordinary activities
- Physical signs such as blushing, sweating, trembling, nausea, and difficulty talking

Treatment

- Behavioral therapy
- Antidepressant therapy

Shyness

Shyness is a form of social anxiety, a fear of what others will think of one's behavior or appearance. Shy people are often excessively self-critical, and they engage in very negative self-talk. Shy people often long to be more outgoing, but their own negative thoughts prevent them from enjoying the social interaction they desire.

Signs and Symptoms

- Rapid heartbeat
- Nervous stomach
- Clammy hands
- Dry mouth or lump in throat
- Trembling muscles

Occurrence

- Approximately 40 to 50 percent of Americans describe themselves as shy.
- Approximately 7 to 13 percent of adults are so shy that their condition interferes seriously with work, school, daily life, or interpersonal relationships.

Causes

- Inherited trait
- Culture and parenting styles
- Stressful events
- Isolation

Treatment

- Shyness classes
- Assertiveness training
- Public speaking
- Cognitive behavioral therapy
- Antidepressant drugs

Post-Traumatic Stress Disorder (PTSD)

PTSD is an anxiety disorder that can develop after exposure to a terrifying event or ordeal in which grave physical harm occurred or was threatened. Traumatic events that may trigger PTSD include violent personal assaults, natural or human-caused disasters, accidents, or military combat.

Signs and Symptoms

Re-experiencing symptoms:
- Flashbacks—reliving the trauma over and over, including physical symptoms like a racing heart or sweating
- Bad dreams
- Frightening thoughts

Avoidance symptoms:
- Staying away from places, events, or objects that are reminders of the experience
- Feeling emotionally numb
- Feeling strong guilt, depression, or worry
- Losing interest in activities that were enjoyable in the past
- Having trouble remembering the dangerous event

Hyperarousal symptoms:
- Being easily startled
- Feeling tense or "on edge"
- Having difficulty sleeping and/or having angry outbursts

Treatment

- Psychotherapy ("talk" therapy)
- Exposure therapy
- Medications

Cutting and Self-harm

Self-injury (self-harm, self-mutilation, cutting) can be defined as the attempt to deliberately cause harm to one's own body and the injury is usually severe enough to cause tissue damage. This is not a conscious attempt at suicide. These are often ways to express deep distress and cope with painful memories.

Signs and Symptoms
- Unexplained wounds
- Indications of depression
- Frequent "accidents"
- Changes in eating habits
- Covering up

Treatment
- Choose a social worker, trauma therapist, psychologist, or psychiatrist who is trained in dealing with self-injury.

What to do when you feel like cutting yourself or self-harming
- **Deal with anger.** Try running, dancing fast, screaming, punching a pillow, throwing something, or ripping something apart.
- **Cope with emotional numbness.** Squeeze ice cubes, hold a package of frozen food, take a very cold shower, or chew something with a very strong taste, like chili peppers, raw ginger root, or a grapefruit peel.
- **Calm yourself.** Take a bubble bath, do deep breathing, write in a journal, draw, or practice yoga.
- **See "blood."** You can draw a red ink line where you would usually cut yourself, in addition to the other suggestions above.

Models of Therapeutic Change

The Behavioral Model

The behavioral model focuses on what people do—their overt behavior—rather than on brain structures and chemistry or on thoughts and consciousness. This model regards psychological problems as bad habits. Behaviorists analyze behavior in terms of stimulus, response, and reinforcement. Behavioral therapy focuses on changing the behavior by adapting a new, healthier habit. This treatment mode also uses exposure therapy, in which the person is exposed to his or her fear.

The Biological Model

The biological model emphasizes that the mind's activity depends entirely on an organic structure, the brain, whose composition is genetically determined. It focuses on genetic evidence and chemicals in the brain that influence our moods and mental health.

Cognitive Model

The cognitive model emphasizes the effect of ideas on behavior and feeling. This model believes that behavior results from complicated attitudes, expectations, and motives rather than simple, immediate reinforcements. It focuses on changing the way a person thinks about the feared situation.

Diet

Nutrition research has shown positive results that a clean diet can play a key role in the onset as well as severity and duration of mental disorders. Serotonin is a neurotransmitter that helps regulate sleep and appetite, mediate moods, and inhibit pain. Your gastrointestinal tract is where 95 percent of your serotonin is produced, in which millions of nerve cells, or neurons guide your emotions. Thus, the bacteria in your gut play an essential role in your health. Studies have shown that when people take probiotics their anxiety levels, perception of stress, and mental outlook improve. Other studies have compared "traditional" diets, like the Mediterranean diet and the traditional Japanese diet, to a typical "Western" diet and have shown that the risk of depression is 2 to 35 percent lower in those who eat a traditional diet. Scientists account for this difference because these traditional diets tend to be high in vegetables, fruits, unprocessed grains, fish and seafood, and modest amounts of lean meats. They avoid all processed and refined carbohdyrates and sugars, and fermented foods rebalance your gut like kombucha tea, miso, sauerkraut, kimchi, and kefir.

Ketogenic diet is effective in treating children with epilepsy. A ketogenic diet is high in fat and very low in carbohydrates. Such a diet can be quite hard to sustain long term though. The idea of the ketogenic diet is to switch the main fuel of the brain from glucose (sugar) to ketones, which are produced when fat is broken down.

> *Seek a Registered Dietitian before going on such a diet.*

Some research has shown that people with ADHD have lower levels of omega-3 fatty acids or may not be able to tolerate gluten. Gluten is a protein found in wheat, rye, and barley. Omega-3 fatty acids may also keep us mentally more stable. Omega-3 fatty acids can be found in oily fish such as cod, salmon, and mackerel. They can also be found in plant sources such as flaxseed and walnuts.

Diets that exclude specific foods thought to be harmful are called **elimination** diets. One such diet for ADHD is the Feingold diet that avoids foods containing synthetic food colors and artificial sweeteners, such as aspartame and preservatives. The Feingold diet also cuts out foods containing salicylic acid. Examples include some apples, red grapes, berries, mushrooms, cucumbers, and tomatoes. Some nuts and spices also have high salicylic acid content. Foods allowed in the Feingold diet include fruits such as banana, grapefruit, pears, and pineapples. Other food allowed include beef, lamb, plain bread, some cereals, milk, eggs, and vitamins that do not contain artificial coloring.

Exercise Therapy

Exercise is not only good for your health, it also can help you reduce depression. A recent study looked at exercise alone in treating mild to moderate depression. The researchers studied adults aged 20 to 45, finding that depressive symptoms were reduced almost 50 percent in individuals who participated in 30-minute aerobic exercise sessions three to five times a week.

Relaxation Techniques

Relaxation techniques help individuals develop the ability to more effectively cope with the stresses that contribute to anxiety, as well as with some of the physical symptoms of anxiety. The techniques taught include breathing retraining and exercise.

The Role of Sleep

Insomnia refers to both the inability to fall asleep, and a broken and restless sleep with early waking. Getting enough sleep is essential to having a healthy body, mind, and spirit. Sleep restores our bodies—it's when many important body functions occur, including tissue regeneration, muscle building, fat metabolism, blood sugar and insulin regulation, and time for conscious and unconscious mind communication. A baby needs 14 to 15 hours of sleep per day, and an adult needs 7 to 9 hours.

Effects of Chronic Sleep Deprivation

- Premature aging
- Obesity, diabetes (type 2) by increasing blood sugar
- Cortisol secretion

How to Get a Good Night's Sleep

- Regulate your body clock.
- Create a conductive sleep environment.
- Don't have caffeine, nicotine, or spicy food at night.
- Finish eating at least two hours before sleep.
- Limit computer and TV use before bed—soothing music and calm books are better choices.
- Meditation, visualization, and yoga can help with relaxation.
- Write in a journal.

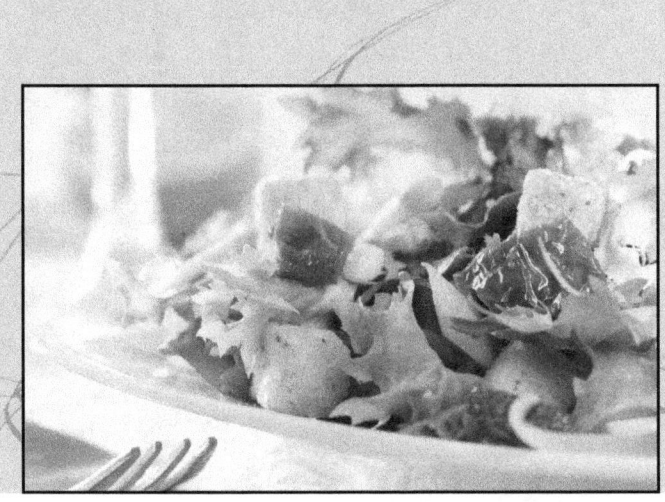

Chapter 4
THE TRUTH ABOUT FOOD

Let food be your medicine.

—Hippocrates

Food is among the most important things that people buy throughout their lives, and yet most people don't bother to take the time to find out exactly what is in the food they buy and consume, where it comes from, or what chemical preservatives might have been added to it. All of the food that a person eats enters the body and becomes part of that person, thereby becoming a major determinant of the person's health. Food affects whether a person is thin or fat, strong or weak, energetic or sluggish, and whether the person will die at a young age or live a long and healthy life. Americans today are bombarded with a vast array of choices and all too often make the mistake of buying food that is toxic. Much of the food produced and sold in the United States is contaminated by toxins, especially in the form of pesticides. In addition, harmful bacteria often enter the food supply from the ways the food is grown, harvested, and processed.

Nutrition

The Six Classes of Nutrients

Macronutrients

- Carbohydrates
- Lipids
- Proteins
- Water

Micronutrients

- Vitamins
- Minerals

▮ *Carbohydrates, lipids, and protein contain calories.*

Calorie (kcal): Amount of heat required to raise temp of 1 kg water 1° C. Calories measure the amount of energy that is released when a specific amount of food is burned.

How Many Calories Do I Need?

Multiply your current weight by the following activity conditions:

    14 if you are sedentary

    15 if you exercise 3 times per week; 40 min.

    16 if you exercise 5 to 7 times per week; 40–60 min.

Weight _____ × Activity level _____ = _____ calories/ day

Remember, regardless of whether you consume carbohydrates, protein, or fat, if you take in more calories than your body requires, your body will convert the excess to fat.

Energy Balance

Body fat is a storage tank for energy; to burn body fat you must release energy from storage.

Energy In = Energy Out + /– Fat Storage

1. Energy In > Energy Out = Weight gain
2. Energy In < Energy Out = Weight loss
3. Energy In = Energy Out = Weight maintenance
   - 1 lb. of fat = 3,500 kcals, so if you want to lose 1 lb. of fat per week you need to cut out 500 calories from your daily intake. (500 calories × 7 days = 3,500 calories = 1 lb. fat)

Energy (Calories) Is Needed to Support Three Major Processes

1. Basal (or resting) metabolism
2. Physical activity
3. Growth

Basal metabolism: The sum total of all the chemical activities of the cells necessary to sustain life, exclusive of voluntary activities—that is, the ongoing activities of the cells when the body is at rest.

Basal metabolic rate (BMR): The rate at which the body spends energy to support its basal metabolism. The BMR accounts for the largest component of a person's daily energy (calorie) needs.

Factors That Affect Metabolism

- Exercise
- Age
- Height

- Yo-yo dieting
- Stimulants
- Frequent meals

How Many Meals Should You Eat Each Day?

Metabolism goes up *only* when you eat consistently all day. You should eat small meals every three hours; divide your total daily calories by 5 to get the number of calories per each meal. For example: 2,000 total daily cal / 5 meals = 400 cal/meal.

Total calories _____ / 5 meals = _____

Goal: Eat five to six small meals per day.

Calorie Values of Common Nutrients

Carbohydrates: 4 calories per gram

Fats (lipids): 9 calories per gram

Proteins: 4 calories per gram

Alcohols: 7 calories per gram

Vitamins, minerals, and water: 0 calories per gram

Acceptable Macronutrient Distribution Ranges (AMDR)[72]

Carbohydrates: 45–65 percent of total daily calories

Fats (lipids): 20–35 percent of total daily calories

Proteins: 10–35 percent of total daily calories

Estimated Calories

Food	Calories	Serving Size
Grains	100	1 slice bread; 1/3 bagel; 1 cup cooked pasta, rice
Dairy	100	1 c. skim, 1% milk; 6 oz. plain yogurt; 1 oz. cheese
Fruit	75	1 piece whole fruit; 1 c. sliced fruit; 6 oz. juice
Food	**Calories**	**Serving Size**
Vegetables	25	4 c. salad greens; 1/2 c. carrots, potatoes; 1 c. vegetables
Protein	150	3 oz. fish, poultry, meat; 3/4 c. tofu; 2 eggs; 2/3 c. cooked beans; 1 oz. nuts
Fat	45	1 tsp oil, margarine, butter; 1 Tbsp dressing; 1/7 of avocado
Goodies	100	1/2 c. frozen yogurt; 3 Tbsp ice cream; 4 oz. wine; 2 1/2 oz. mixed drink; 3/4 of a chocolate bar; 2 Tbsp sugar

Some Favorite Meals	Calories
1 c. lasagna; mac & cheese; chili	340
1 c. chicken shrimp w/broccoli	265
1 slice cheese pizza	300
6 pieces sushi roll	225
1 tuna sandwich (homemade)	325
6–8 cheese nachos (no meat)	345
Big Mac & large fries (McDonald's)	1,090
Original Whopper w/cheese, large fries (Burger King)	1,300
KFC 3-piece chicken meal	1,010
Porterhouse steak	1,100
Medium movie popcorn	1,100
Chinese kung pao chicken	1,620

Water

Functions

Water is the most important environmental substance essential to human life. It makes up about 80 percent of the liquid substance of all cells. Approximately 40 to 60 percent of a person's body weight consists of water. Water makes up about 72 percent of the weight of muscle tissue and only 20 to 25 percent of the weight of fat.

- Essential for body temperature regulation
- Transports nutrients and wastes in the body
- Serves as a medium for every enzymatic and chemical reaction
- Maintains blood volume
- Is critical for nerve impulse conduction
- Yields no energy
- Even small amounts of dehydration can impair performance

Goal

64 ounces/day

Proteins

Functions

Proteins are critical for growth, maintenance, and repair of muscles, bones, blood, hair, and fingernails. They are key to synthesis of enzymes, hormones, and antibodies and provide essential amino acids.

Characteristics

- 4 calories per gram
- 22 amino acids total; 9 essential amino acids (must be included through food)
- Complete versus incomplete proteins; may come from animal sources (complete proteins) or plant (incomplete)

- Too much protein = health problems: must be processed (kidneys may be overtaxed)
- In animal form, proteins are associated with saturated fats and cholesterol, heart disease, and osteoporosis.
- You need more protein when you are growing, sick, or injured, have undergone surgery, are pregnant, or are engaging in strenuous exercise.

Smart, Lean Proteins

- Lean chicken—white meat (no skin)
- Fish
- Turkey (white meat)
- Nuts
- Tofu
- Skim milk, low-fat cheese, yogurt
- Egg whites

Goal

0.8–1.0 grams per kilogram

Carbohydrates

Functions

- Provides our brains and body with glucose

Characteristics

4 calories per gram

Simple Carbohydrates (Sugars)

↑blood sugar→↑insulin→fat storage, moodiness, cravings, hunger→quickly absorbs sugar→↓blood sugar.

Simple sugars break down rapidly and the rise in blood sugar provides a quick burst of energy, often followed by a crash.

Monosaccharides (simple sugars) have only single sugar unit in their structure. Monosaccharide units can combine together to form **disaccharides** (containing two sugar units) or **polysaccharides** as starch (containing several sugar units).

- **Glucose**—also known as grape sugar, corn sugar, starch sugar and blood sugar. Found in fruits, vegetables, honey, and starch.
- **Sucrose**—also known as table sugar; is made of glucose and fructose molecules. Found in sugar beets and sugar cane and processed food.
- **Fructose**—also known as fruit sugar. Naturally available in honey; fruits such as apples, pears, grapes, peach, banana, apricot, berries, dried fruits, and melons; and vegetables such as beets, sweet potatoes, sweet corn, carrot, red pepper, onion, yam, and sugar cane.
- **Lactose**—also known as milk sugar. The body breaks lactose down into galactose and glucose.

How to Calculate How Much Sugar Is in a Product

Example: A 20-ounce bottle of Coca-Cola contains about 16.87 teaspoons of sugar. You get this by multiplying 27 (the number of grams of sugar in a serving) by 2.5 (the number of servings in a bottle), which = 67.5 grams of sugar in a bottle. One teaspoon = 4 grams, so divide 67.5 grams by 4 to get the teaspoons of sugar.

What Is Lactose Intolerance?

Lactose intolerance is the inability or insufficient ability to digest lactose. It's caused by a deficiency of the enzyme lactase, which is produced by the cells lining the small intestine. Lactase breaks down lactose, glucose, and galactose, which are then absorbed into the bloodstream. Lactose intolerance is NOT a milk allergy. Milk allergy is a reaction by the body's immune system to one or more milk proteins and can be life-threatening when just a small amount of milk or milk product is consumed.

Symptoms of lactose intolerance:
- abdominal pain
- abdominal bloating
- gas
- diarrhea
- nausea

Two tests are commonly used to measure the digestion of lactose:
- **Hydrogen Breath Test.** The person drinks a lactose-loaded beverage and then the breath is analyzed at regular intervals to measure the amount of hydrogen.
- **Stool Acidity Test.** The stool acidity test is used for infants and young children to measure the amount of acid in the stool.

Treatment

People with lactose intolerance should choose milk products with lower levels of lactose than regular milk, such as yogurt and hard cheese. Lactose-free and lactose-reduced milk and milk products are available at most supermarkets. These products are identical to regular milk except that the lactase enzyme has been added.

Complex Carbohydrates
- Fiber and starch
- Healthier than simple carbohydrates
- Examples: vegetables, grains, cereals, nuts, beans

Goal
- Get at least 130 grams/day to support brain function.
- Limit added sugars to no more than 25 percent of total daily calories.
- Get at least three servings of whole grain per day.

Smart Carbohydrates

- 100% Whole grains
- Oats, wheat, barley, rye, quinoa, couscous
- Brown rice
- Baked potato (with skin)
- Whole-wheat pasta
- Beans
- Whole fruit, *not* juice

Fiber (20–35 g/day)

- Proposed definition (IOM Report, 2001): "consists of non-digestible food plant carbohydrates and lignin"
  Fiber terms:
  - **Soluble:** Makes you feel full; lowers blood cholesterol; beans, oats, carrots, peas, apples, citrus, barley, rice, etc.
  - **Insoluble:** Removes toxins; prevents hemorrhoids, increases elimination; wheat bran

  Both types decrease risk of diabetes, obesity, and certain cancers.

Goal

- *Men:* 38 grams of fiber/day; 50+ years: 30 grams
- *Women:* 25 grams of fiber/day; 50+ years: 21 grams

Fats

Functions

- Carry and help with absorption of the fat-soluble vitamins A, D, E, and K
- Protect organs from injury
- Regulate body temperature
- Play an important role in growth and development

Characteristics

- 9 calories per gram
- Saturated versus unsaturated fats versus trans-fats

Goal

20–35 percent of total daily calories

Saturated Fats

- Increase cholesterol
- Increase LDL
- Increase risk of heart disease
- Increase risk of colon, prostate cancer

  Sources of saturated fat include:
  - Meat, poultry
  - Egg yolks
  - Butter
  - Dairy products
  - Coconut
  - Palm oil

Trans-Fats

- "Partially hydrogenated" or "shortening"
- Produced during hydrogenation of fats in manufacturing
- Increase risk of heart disease
- "Eating plastic"
  - Margarine
  - Baked goods
  - Cookies
  - Crackers
  - Peanut butter
  - Pancake mix

Polyunsaturated Fats

- Lower total cholesterol
- Decrease HDL
  - Omega 3's (fish, walnuts, almonds, flaxseeds)
- Decrease blood clotting and inflammation
- Decrease triglycerides
- Decrease blood pressure
- Decrease risk of heart attacks, strokes, and some cancer
- Slightly increase risk of cancer if Omega 6 consumption is greater than Omega 3 consumption
- Omega 6's (vegetable oils)

Monounsaturated Fats

- Decrease total cholesterol and LDL
- Decrease blood pressure
- Decrease triglycerides
- Decrease risk of heart attacks, strokes, and some cancers
  - Olive oil
  - Peanut oil
  - Avocados
  - Canola

Cholesterol

- Made in the liver
- Only found in animal products
- We need it, but high intake may cause CVD; saturated fats are worse
- Transported in water-soluble vehicles:
  - Very-low-density lipoproteins
  - Low-density lipoproteins
  - High-density lipoproteins

Goal

Less than 200 mg daily

Smart Fats

- Olive oil, olives
- Canola
- Fish
- Nuts
- Avocado
- Flaxseeds

Nuts

In 2003, the U.S. Food and Drug Administration (FDA) approved this "qualified" health claim on a package label for nuts:

> "Scientific evidence suggests but does not prove that eating 1.5 ounces per day of most nuts, as part of a diet low in saturated fat and cholesterol, may reduce the risk of heart disease."[73]

A "qualified" health claim means the FDA evaluated the data and determined "though there is scientific evidence to support this claim, the evidence is not conclusive." A qualified health claim is issued by the FDA when it is determined that consumers will benefit from more information on a dietary supplement or conventional food label concerning diet and health even though the claim is based on "somewhat settled science rather than just on the standard of significant scientific agreement, as long as the claims do not mislead the consumers." For more information about qualified health claims, go to: www.cfsan.fda.gov/~dms/labqhcqa.html.

According to the FDA, "Types of nuts eligible for this claim are restricted to almonds, hazelnuts, peanuts, pecans, some pine nuts, pistachio nuts and walnuts. Types of nuts on which the health claim may be placed is restricted to those nuts that were specifically included in the health claim petition, but that do not exceed 4 g saturated fat per 50 g of nuts."

Though nuts are a higher-fat food, it is a mostly heart-healthy unsaturated fat and may help lower low-density lipoproteins (LDL or bad cholesterol).

Vegetarian Diets

- *Vegans* exclude all animal products, the most restrictive type of vegetarian diet.
- *Lacto-ovo* vegetarians only exclude meat.
- A modified vegetarian diet promotes health and weight management.
- Legumes and soy have particular health benefits.
- Vitamin deficiencies (protein, vitamin B_{12}, iron, calcium, zinc) can result from a careless vegetarian diet.
- Health benefits of a vegetarian diet include: lower cholesterol, lower body fat, lower blood pressure, and lower risk of some cancers.

What Are Vitamins?

Functions

- Help put proteins, fats, and carbohydrates to use
- Essential for regulating growth, maintaining tissue, and releasing energy from food
- Involved in the manufacture of blood cells, hormones, and other compounds

Characteristics

- *Fat-soluble*: vitamins A, D, E, and K; stored in the liver; toxic in high amounts
- *Water-soluble*: B vitamins (eight total) and vitamin C

Antioxidants

- Vitamins C and E and beta-carotene, carotenoids, and flavonoids are antioxidants.
- Antioxidants destroy free radicals in your body.

Free radicals: Result of normal metabolism, pollution, smoking, radiation, and stress

Minerals

Functions

- Help build bones and teeth
- Aid in muscle function
- Help our nervous system transmit messages

Characteristics

- 16 minerals
- *Major:* sodium, potassium, chloride, calcium, phosphorus, magnesium, and sulfur
- *Trace:* iron, zinc, selenium, molybdenum, iodine, copper, manganese, fluoride, and chromium

Goal

- Dietary reference intakes: To find out the dietary reference intake for vitamins and minerals, go to www.iom.edu/.

Phytonutrients

Phytonutrients are substances plants use to defend themselves against disease attacks. These generally colorful compounds, like the lycopene in tomatoes, appear to help humans fend off serious ailments, including cancer and heart disease. They are found naturally in fruits and vegetables.

	Found In	Function		
Vitamin A Retinol	liver, fortified milk (Retinol form—see following for carotene sources)	Essential for eyes, skin, and the proper function of the immune system. Helps maintain hair, bones, and teeth.	**Deficiency causes:** night blindness; reduced hair growth in children; loss of appetite; dry, rough skin; lowered resistance to infection; dry eyes **Overdose causes:** headaches; blurred vision; fatigue; diarrhea; irregular periods; joint and bone pain; dry, cracked skin; rashes; loss of hair; vomiting; liver damage	
Beta Carotene (pro-vitamin A) (see also vitamin A)	carrots, squash, broccoli, green leafy vegetables	Antioxidant. Converted to vitamin A in the body. (See vitamin A.)		**Claim:** The antioxidant properties of this nutrient may be a factor in reducing the risk of certain forms of cancer.

	Found In	**Function**		
Vitamin D	egg yolk, milk. Exposure to sun enables body to make its own vitamin D.	Helps build and maintain teeth and bones. Enhances calcium absorption.	**Deficiency causes:** rickets in children; bone softening in adults; osteoporosis **Overdose causes:** calcium deposits in organs; fragile bones; renal and cardio-vascular damage	
Vitamin E	corn or cottonseed oil, butter, brown rice, soybean oil, vegetable oils such as corn, cottonseed, or soybean, nuts, wheat germ	Antioxidant. Helps form red blood cells, muscles, and other tissues. Preserves fatty acids.	**Deficiency causes:** rare, seen primarily in premature or low-birth-weight babies or children who do not absorb fat properly; causes nerve abnormalities **Overdose causes:** unknown	**Claim:** The antioxidant properties of this nutrient may be a factor in reducing the risk of certain forms of cancer.
Vitamin K	green vegetables, liver, also made by intestinal bacteria	Needed for normal blood clotting.	**Deficiency causes:** defective blood coagulation **Overdose:** jaundice in infants	

Water-soluble vitamins are not stored in the body and can therefore be consumed daily.

	Found In	**Function**		
Thiamine Vitamin B$_1$	sunflower seeds, pork, whole and enriched grains, dried beans	Necessary for carbohydrate metabolism and muscle coordination. Promotes proper nerve function.	**Deficiency causes:** anxiety; hysteria; depression; muscle cramps; loss of appetite; in extreme cases beriberi (mostly in alcoholics) **Overdose causes:** unknown, although excess of one B vitamin may cause deficiency of others	
Riboflavin Vitamin B$_2$	liver, milk, spinach, enriched noodles, mushrooms	Needed for metabolism of all foods and the release of energy to cells. Essential to the functioning of vitamin B$_6$ and niacin.	**Deficiency causes:** cracks and sores around the mouth and nose; visual problems **Overdose causes:** see vitamin B$_1$	

	Found In	**Function**	
Niacin Vitamin B_3 Niacin is converted to niacinamide in the body.	mushrooms, bran, tuna, chicken, beef, peanuts, enriched grains	Needed in many enzymes that convert food to energy. Helps maintain a healthy digestive tract and nervous system. In very large doses, lowers cholesterol (large doses should only be taken under the advice of a physician).	**Deficiency causes:** in extreme cases, pellagra, a disease characterized by dermatitis, diarrhea, and mouth sores **Overdose causes:** hot flashes; ulcers; liver disorders; high blood sugar and uric acid; cardiac arrythmias
Pantothenic Acid Vitamin B_5	abundant in animal tissues, whole-grain cereals, and legumes	Converts food to molecular forms. Needed to manufacture adrenal hormones and chemicals that regulate nerve function.	**Deficiency causes:** unclear in humans **Overdose causes:** see Vitamin B_1
Vitamin B_6 Pyridoxine	animal protein foods, spinach, broccoli, bananas	Needed for protein metabolism and absorption, carbohydrate metabolism. Helps form red blood cells. Promotes nerve and brain function.	**Deficiency causes:** anemia; irritability; patches of itchy, scaling skin; convulsions **Overdose causes:** nerve damage
Vitamin B_{12} Cyanocobalamin	found almost exclusively in animal products	Builds genetic material. Helps form red blood cells.	**Deficiency causes:** pernicious anemia; nerve damage. (Note: Deficiency rare except in strict vegetarians, the elderly, or people with malabsorption disorders.) **Overdose causes:** see vitamin B_1
Biotin	cheese, egg yolk, cauliflower, peanut butter	Needed for metabolism of glucose and formation of certain fatty acids. Essential for proper body chemistry.	**Deficiency causes:** seborrhic dermatitis in infants; rare in adults, but can be induced by consuming large amounts of egg whites—anorexia, nausea, vomiting, dry scaly skin **Overdose causes:** see vitamin B_1

	Found In	**Function**		
Folic Acid (Folacin)	green leafy vegetables, orange juice, organ meats, sprouts	Essential for the manufacture of genetic material as well as protein metabolism and red blood cell formation.	**Deficiency causes:** impaired cell division; anemia; diarrhea; gastrointestinal upsets; spina bifida **Overdose causes:** convulsions in epileptics; may mask pernicious anemia (see vitamin B_{12} deficiency)	**Claim:** Adequate amounts of this nutrient in the first stage of pregnancy may reduce the risks of neural tube birth defects.
Vitamin C Ascorbic Acid	citrus fruits, strawberries, broccoli, green peppers	Antioxidant. Helps bind cells together and strengthens blood vessel walls. Helps maintain healthy gums. Aids in the absorption of iron.	**Deficiency causes:** muscle weakness; bleeding gums; easy bruising; in extreme cases, scurvy. **Overdose causes:** unknown	**Claim:** The antioxidant properties of this nutrient may be a factor in reducing the risk of certain forms of cancer. May reduce the effects of the common cold.

Minerals found in organic products are essential for body functions.

	Found In	Function		
Calcium	milk, yogurt, cheese, sardines, broccoli, turnip greens	Helps build strong bones and teeth. Promotes muscle and nerve function. Helps blood to clot. Helps activate enzymes needed to convert food to energy.	**Deficiency causes:** rickets in children; osteomalacia (soft bones) and osteoporosis in adults. **Overdose causes:** constipation, kidney stones, calcium deposits in body tissues; hinders absorption of iron and other minerals	
Phosphorus	chicken, breast milk, lentils, egg yolks, nuts, cheese	With calcium builds bones and teeth. Needed for metabolism, body chemistry, nerve and muscle function.	**Deficiency causes:** (rare) weakness; bone pain; anorexia **Overdose causes:** hinders body's absorption of calcium	
Magnesium	spinach, beef greens, broccoli, tofu, popcorn, cashews, wheat bran	Activates enzymes needed to release energy in body. Needed by cells for genetic material and bone growth.	**Deficiency causes:** nausea; irritability; muscle weakness; twitching; cramps; cardiac arrhythmias **Overdose causes:** nausea; vomiting; low blood pressure; nervous system disorders	**Warning:** Overdose can be fatal to people with kidney disease.

	Found In	**Function**	
Potassium	peanuts, bananas, orange juice, green beans, mushrooms, oranges, broccoli, sunflower seeds	Helps maintain regular fluid balance. Needed for nerve and muscle function.	Deficiency causes: nausea; anorexia; muscle weakness; irritability (occurs most often in persons with prolonged diarrhea). Overdose causes: rare
Iron (Elemental)	liver, lean meats, kidney beans, enriched bread, raisins. Note: Oxalic acid in spinach hinders iron absorption.	Essential for making hemoglobin, the red substance in blood that carries oxygen to body cells.	Deficiency causes: skin pallor; weakness; fatigue; headaches; shortness of breath (all signs of iron-deficiency anemia). Overdose causes: toxic buildup in liver and, in rare instances, the heart
Zinc	oysters, shrimp, crab, beef, turkey, whole grains, peanuts, beans	Necessary element in more than 100 enzymes that are essential to digestion and metabolism.	Deficiency causes: slow healing of wounds; loss of taste; retarded growth and delayed sexual development in children. Overdose causes: nausea, vomiting; diarrhea; abdominal pain; gastric bleeding
Selenium	adequate amounts are found in seafood, kidney, liver and other meats. Grains and other seeds contain varying amounts depending on the soil content.	Antioxidant. Interacts with vitamin E to prevent breakdown of fats and body chemicals.	Deficiency causes: unknown in humans Overdose causes: fingernail changes, hair loss
Copper	liver and other organ meats, seafood, nuts and seeds	Component of several enzymes, including ones needed to make skin, hair, and other pigments. Stimulates iron absorption. Needed to make red blood cells, connective tissue, and nerve fibers.	Deficiency causes: rare in adults, infants may develop a type of anemia marked by abnormal development of bones, nerve tissue, and lungs Overdose causes: liver disease; vomiting; diarrhea

	Found In	Function	
Manganese	tea, whole grains, and cereal products are the richest dietary sources; adequate amounts are found in fruits and vegetables	Needed for normal tendon and bone structure. Component of some enzymes important in metabolism.	**Deficiency causes:** unknown in humans **Overdose causes:** generally results from inhalation of manganese-containing dust or fumes, not dietary ingestion
Molybdenum	The concentration in food varies depending on the environment in which the food was grown; milk, beans, breads and cereals contribute the highest amounts.	Component of enzymes needed in metabolism. Helps regulate iron storage.	**Deficiency causes:** unknown in humans **Overdose causes:** gout-like joint pain

The Bitter Truth About Fast Food

The fast food industry in the United States makes billions of dollars every year, despite growing concerns about the increasing rates of obesity, even among children, as well as increasing incidences of food poisoning. Studies have shown that Americans currently spend more money on fast food than they do on higher education, cars, personal computers, books, magazines, videos, and CDs. One survey found that 96 percent of young American children could identify Ronald McDonald, and the golden arches that symbolize McDonald's was more widely recognized than the Christian cross.

Fat, Sugar, and Salt

Have you ever wondered why you can't stop at just 10 potato chips? Next thing you know, the entire bag is eaten. Companies use fat, sugar, and salt to addict us. They add these ingredients to make you an addict and to make a lot of profit. These foods are made in a laboratory using many addictive chemicals. Fast food tastes good partly because of added ingredients such as chemicals, "natural" and artificial flavors, and even food coloring. Studies indicate that such additives can have a significant effect on how a person perceives the taste of food. In addition, some of the chemicals added to fast food are actually addictive, which helps explain why many adults who have regularly eaten fast food since they were children cannot simply quit eating it; they actually experience withdrawal symptoms when they go without it. When we eat processed foods compromised of sugars, salts, and fats, we crave more. Our bodies also start to deteriorate.

For these and other reasons, it is important that people carefully read the labels on the foods they choose. The terms "natural flavor" and "artificial flavor" on food labels refer to human-made additives that enhance the taste of most processed foods. Commercials suggesting that people cannot stop after eating just a few potato chips are not far off the mark; it is very difficult for most people to stop because of the addictive ingredients and flavor enhancers that have been added to chips and other similar snacks.

Coloring agents are added to many soft drinks, salad dressings, condiments, chicken dishes, cookies, bread, and other baked products. The Food and Drug Administration (FDA) does not require the manufacturers of food flavorings to disclose the ingredients in the flavorings, as long as all the chemicals they contain are considered by the FDA to be "generally regarded as safe" (GRAS). This lack of a requirement to publicly disclose ingredients enables the manufacturers to maintain the secrecy of their formulas.

Example of a Widespread Coloring Agent

Do you eat strawberry yogurt, milkshakes, or frozen fruit bars? If so, you have probably been eating insects, too. Cochineal extract (also known as carmine or carminic acid) is a dye made from the dried, crushed bodies of the female *Dactylopius coccus*, or cochineal, a small insect that is harvested in Peru, the Canary Islands, Chile, and Mexico. Cochineals eat red cactus berries. The carmine color from the berries accumulates in the bodies of the females and in their unhatched larvae, producing the carmine dye. In addition to yogurt, frozen fruit bars, and milkshakes, some other sweets, fruit fillings, and juice drinks also get their pink color from carmine.

Factory Farming

Most animals raised for food in the United States are raised on factory farms. Many animals are raised in inhumane conditions, injected with steroids and hormones, which thus raise health concerns for the consumer. Factory farming also contributes to the emissions of greenhouse gases, which is responsible for global warming. Cows, through belching and flatulence, emit methane that is 23 times more powerful than carbon dioxide.

Ground Meat

Hamburgers are one of the most popular foods worldwide. The Center for Science in the Public Interest (CSPI) studied 12 years of government data on food-borne illnesses. The consumer advocacy organization says the results point to chicken and ground beef as the riskiest of meats. Ground meat can be made from different animal parts, different types of animals, other ingredients ground in with the meat and therefore has the highest contamination of *E. coli* and salmonella.

Countless cows are needed to produce the millions of hamburgers that are consumed daily throughout the world, and turning that much cattle into such a huge amount of beef meat requires large-scale industrial processes. A huge number of resources are needed to raise cattle, including land resources, water, soybeans, and grain to feed the cattle, which is often produced by chemical intensive-farming. It takes about 2,500 gallons of water and 16 pounds of grain and soybeans to produce just a single pound of hamburger. Multiplying these numbers by the estimated 67 to 69 pounds of beef that an average meat-eating American consumes per year adds up to an enormous amount of resources. In South America, huge areas of tropical rain forests have been cleared to make room for grazing land for cattle. The continuing destruction of rain forests is extinguishing countless and as yet undiscovered species of plants that could be medicinally beneficial to humans, not to mention the increased potential for global warming that rain-forest destruction is creating.

Other Meat Products

According to many scientists and researchers, meat products are becoming increasingly dangerous as a result of the way in which animals are raised and slaughtered. They often are confined to tiny cages crowded together, enabling illnesses and infections to be easily passed from one animal to another. As a result, industrial farms frequently resort to the use of antibiotics to prevent the animals from becoming ill or diseased. It is not uncommon for industrial meat producers to slaughter numerous animals at one time and mix their meat together.

Although hogs produce three times the amount of fecal waste than humans do, hog farms are not required to treat the sewage of their animals. Instead, hog waste is typically stored in large ponds called lagoons.

According to Eric Schlosser, who investigated slaughterhouses for his book and movie *Fast Food Nation*, hog lagoons filled with waste can be as extensive as 20 acres and as deep as 15 feet. Dangerous chemicals, including hydrogen sulfide and ammonia, emanate from the lagoons. Some studies suggest that when humans breathe air polluted with hydrogen sulfide over a certain period of time, permanent damage to the nervous system and the brain can result. Moreover, the liquid waste from the lagoons is regularly sprayed onto fields, where it infests the soil with bacteria and toxins. Groundwater and nearby streams are commonly poisoned by the leakage and the overflowing of hog lagoons, and there are dead zones in the rivers downstream from these factory farms.

The huge slaughterhouses in which the animals are killed are dangerous and disturbing environments as well. The unskilled labor of meatpacking is both dirty and dangerous, and few slaughterhouses are unionized. Many of the workers are recent immigrants and illegal aliens. As for the animals, when cattle are driven through a chute into a slaughterhouse, a worker called a "knocker" shoots each steer in the head with a stun-gun that drives a retractable steel bolt into its brain. Once the animal has fallen lifelessly to the ground, another worker fastens a chain and hook attached to a pulley around one of the steer's rear legs, and the steer is then hauled upside down into the air. A worker called a "sticker" then slits the unconscious animal's throat about once every 10 seconds. The carcass then moves on down the disassembly line past other workers, with chainsaws, hooks, and knives, who carve it up into the parts to be sold for retail. Modern slaughterhouses can process thousands of heads of cattle in one day in this manner, resulting in the production of about 800,000 pounds of hamburger meat. It is entirely possible that the meat in a single fast-food hamburger could have come from dozens or even hundreds of steers.

The waste from the cattle carcasses in a slaughterhouse is melted down, into a mixture of meat and bone meal. This mixture is used to make food for other animals to help them grow larger and more quickly. Animals that are raised for their meat or dairy products are also given growth hormones and steroids so as to maximize their growth and therefore, their market value, in the shortest possible period of time. Large amounts of antibiotics are also used to prevent diseases from spreading throughout a population of overcrowded animals, which has the negative consequence of creating drug-resistant bacteria in humans. Essentially, when humans eat the meat of animals that have been given hormones, steroids, and/or antibiotics, they are ingesting secondhand all of these substances themselves. This too can have harmful effects on the health of humans who eat the meat of these animals, including the potential to cause disease.

Two of the hormones that the meat industry uses, estradiol and zeranol, are likely to have harmful effects on humans, including cancer and hormonal changes. Concerns about these potential health impacts have caused many scientists to doubt the safety of hormone use in meat production.

Poultry litter is another type of animal feed made from biological waste. Poultry litter is a mixture of chicken excrement, spilled feed, dirt, feathers, and everything else that is scooped up from the floors of poultry sheds. Because poultry litter is much less expensive than plant crops are, the cattle industry in the United States feeds approximately one million tons of poultry litter to cattle every year.

Chicken McNuggets

The name "Chicken McNugget" is a bit of an exaggeration. In fact, a chicken McNugget is made up of about 56 percent corn and 38 other ingredients besides chicken. The most disturbing ingredient in Chicken McNuggets is tertiary butylhydroquinone (TBHQ), an antioxidant that is derived from petroleum. TBHQ is either sprayed directly on the nuggets or on the inside of the boxes that they are put into to "help preserve freshness." According to *A Consumer's Dictionary of Food Additives*, TBHQ is a form of butane (i.e., lighter fluid). Still, the FDA allows food processors to use it sparingly in food intended for human consumption. TBHQ can make up no more than 0.02% of the oil in a single nugget of chicken. However, if a person ingests just a single gram of TBHQ, it can cause nausea, vomiting, delirium, a feeling of suffocation, and even the collapse of the person. If a person ingests 5 grams of TBHQ, it can be fatal.

In addition to TBHQ, the fat content of chicken nuggets is a concern. Between 50 and 60 percent of the calories in most chicken nuggets comes from fat. The popularity of high-fat, highly processed fast foods, including chicken nuggets, is one of the reasons why the percentage of American children who are overweight has tripled in the past 20 years. Following is McDonalds's own nutritional breakdown of a typical serving of Chicken McNuggets:

Ingredients:

White boneless chicken, water, food starch-modified, salt, chicken flavor (autolyzed yeast extract, salt, wheat starch, natural flavoring (botanical source), safflower oil, dextrose, citric acid, rosemary), sodium phosphates, seasoning (canola oil, mono- and diglycerides, natural extractives of rosemary). Battered and breaded with: water, enriched flour (bleached wheat flour, niacin, reduced iron, thiamin mononitrate, riboflavin, folic acid), yellow corn flour, food starch-modified, salt, leavening (baking soda, sodium acid pyrophosphate, sodium aluminum phosphate, monocalcium phosphate, calcium lactate), spices, wheat starch, whey, corn starch. Prepared in vegetable oil ((may contain one of the following: canola oil, corn oil, soybean oil, hydrogenated soybean oil, partially hydrogenated soybean oil, *partially hydrogenated corn oil with TBHQ and citric acid added to preserve freshness), dimethylpolysiloxane added as an antifoaming agent). CONTAINS: WHEAT AND MILK

Nutrition Facts:

Serving size: 6 nuggets
Calories: 310
Fat calories: 180
Fat: 20 grams
Carbohydrates: 18 grams
Protein: 15 grams
Percentage fat: 58%
*partially hydrogenated = trans fat
(Source: McDonald's USA Ingredients http://www.mcdonalds.com/)

What You Can Do

Clearly, millions of animals caught within the process of factory farming suffer. If you don't want to be a part of this, you can switch to free-range or organic meat products. Organic chicken meat, especially meat from chickens raised on farms near where you live, is the most healthful choice. Organic chickens are better fed, less exposed to pesticides and harmful chemicals, and exposed to some sunlight, all of which makes them more healthful for human consumption. If you like chicken nuggets, stop eating the fast-food version and, instead, make them yourself and help improve your health. A recipe for healthful chicken nuggets is provided below.

Make Your Own Healthful Chicken Nuggets:

Ingredients:

- 1 cup dry bread crumbs
- ¼ cup parmesan cheese

- 2 tsp dried oregano
- 2 tsp dried basil
- 1 tsp paprika
- ½ tsp dried thyme
- 1½ lb. boneless, skinless chicken breasts, cup into 2-inch cubes
- 1 tbsp olive oil

Instructions:

1. Preheat oven to 350 degrees.
2. In a large plastic bag, mix together all the ingredients except the chicken and oil.
3. After mixing together the ingredients, add the chicken cubes to the plastic bag and shake well.
4. On a nonstick cookie sheet, place the chicken cubes.
5. Either lightly spray olive oil from a bottle or sprinkle olive oil over the chicken.
6. Bake the chicken cubes for about 10 minutes, or until they are fully cooked.

Nutritional Information:

Calories: 239
Calories from Fat: 64
Total Fat: 7 g
Cholesterol: 71 mg
Sodium: 275 mg
Carbohydrate: 13 g
Dietary Fiber: 1 g
Sugar: 1 g
Protein: 29 g

McDonald's French Fries

In June of 2002, the McDonald's corporation was forced to pay $10 million to Hindu and vegetarian groups in the United States because it had misled the public about its French fries being vegetarian. Hindus do not eat beef for religious reasons. The groups of Hindus and vegetarians involved in the lawsuit against McDonald's had eaten French fries that had been pre-cooked in beef tallow, which McDonald's had described as "natural flavoring."

McDonald's described the production of its French fries on its website in January of 2003 in the following way: "A small amount of beef flavoring is added during potato processing at the plant. After the potatoes are washed and steam- peeled, they are cut, blanched, dried, par-fried, and frozen. It is during the par-frying process at the plant that the natural flavoring is used. These fries are then shipped to our U.S. restaurants. Our French fries are cooked in vegetable oil at our restaurants."

In September of 2002, McDonald's pledged to start using a new oil that would contain half the level of harmful trans-fatty acids in its French fries as before. However, the company delayed those plans, citing product quality and customer satisfaction as priorities while testing of new oils continued. As a result of new and improved testing, in 2006, it was found that McDonald's French fries contained a third more trans fats than had previously been thought. This finding was based on the results of a new testing method that the company had begun to use the previous year. The conclusion is that the amount of potentially artery-clogging trans fat in a large serving of French fries is actually 8 grams, not the previously reported 6 grams, meaning that the total amount of fat contained in a large serving is actually 30 grams, not 25.

Concerns About Acrylamide

Acrylamide is a chemical that is produced during the frying, baking, or grilling of nearly all carbohydrate-rich foods, especially fast-food French fries. Many scientists believe that acrylamide can cause nervous tremors in people who ingest the chemical in high amounts, and it has been associated with birth defects, male infertility, and cancer in lab animals. California's attorney general has joined a suit against McDonald's and other fast-food chains to require them to label their French fries accordingly. Following is McDonalds's own nutritional breakdown of a typical serving of its French fries:

Ingredients:

Potatoes, vegetable oil (partially hydrogenated soybean oil, natural beef flavor (wheat and milk derivatives)*, citric acid (preservative), dextrose, sodium acid pyrophosphate (maintain color), dimethylpolysiloxane (antifoaming agent)), salt. Prepared in vegetable oil ((may contain one of the following: canola oil, corn oil, soybean oil, hydrogenated soybean oil, partially hydrogenated soybean oil, partially hydrogenated corn oil with TBHQ and citric acid added to preserve freshness), dimethylpolysiloxane added as an antifoaming agent). (Natural beef flavor contains hydrolyzed wheat and hydrolyzed milk as starting ingredients.)
*CONTAINS: WHEAT AND MILK

Nutrition Facts (Serving Size: 1 large order)

Total Fat: 30.0 g
Saturated Fat: 6.0 g; 46% of DV
Carbohydrates: 70.0 g
Sodium: 330 mg
Calories from Fat: 270
Calories: 570
Protein: 6.0 g
Source: McDonald's USA Ingredients (http://www.mcdonalds.com/)

Make Your Own Healthful French Fries

Ingredients:

potatoes
salt
canola oil

1. Peel and slice potatoes, then place them in a mixing bowl with cold water and ice cubes. Soak for 30 minutes. Preheat oven to 400°F.

2. After soaking the potatoes, drain them and then pat them dry with a paper towel.

3. Place the potatoes and salt in a plastic zipper bag. Spray the potatoes for about 3 seconds with canola oil, and then seal the plastic zipper bag. Shake to coat the potatoes well with the oil and salt.

4. Carefully place the potatoes on a non-stick cookie sheet so that they don't touch one another. Spray lightly with canola oil.

5. Place the cookie sheet in the oven and allow the potatoes to bake for about 7 minutes. Turn the potatoes at least twice, cooking for about 7 minutes after each turn. The total cooking time is 20–25 minutes.

Nutrition Facts:

Calories: 86
Total Fat: 0 g
Saturated Fat: 0 g
Trans Fat: 0 g
Cholesterol: 0 mg
Sodium: 297 mg
Total Carbohydrates: 20 g
Dietary Fiber: 2 g
Sugars: 1 g
Protein: 2 g

Go Meatless on Mondays:

Going meatless just once a week may help reduce your carbon footprint by saving resources like fresh water and fossil fuel. It will also have a significant benefit to your health if you replace the meat with vegetarian sources of protein like fish, nuts, beans, organic soy, and quinoa.

Fish

Fish is a high quality protein, low in fat and high in Omega-3s and Vitamin D, which is great for your heart and brain.

Omega-3 Fatty Acids:

- Lowers blood pressure and reduces the risk of sudden death, heart attack, abnormal heart rhythms, and strokes
- Helps healthy brain function and infant development of vision and nerves during pregnancy
- Decreases the risk of depression, ADHD, Alzheimer's disease, dementia, and diabetes
- Reduces inflammation and the risk of arthritis

Fish and seafood farming is the fastest growing sector of food production in the world and one of the fastest growing threats to marine environments and their native species. There are health and food-safety concerns about human consumption of farm-bred fish. Fish that have been farmed often are given large doses of antibiotics to protect them from diseases. They also are exposed to a number of pesticides that kill parasites and body fungi, all of which accumulate in the tissues of the fish. When people eat this fish, they also ingest traces of the pesticides, which can remain in the internal organs.

The most common farm-raised fish include catfish, salmon, trout, and shrimp. When you buy fish, make sure to read the labels or ask an employee whether the fish is wild or farm-raised. Choose wild fish to help protect your health.

Mercury pollution is another concern about human consumption of fish. Mercury from coal-fired power plants is absorbed into the air, deposited in bodies of water through natural weather processes, and enters the skin of fish. The fish that are most commonly contaminated with mercury include tuna, sea bass, farm-raised salmon, swordfish, shark, tilefish, and king mackerel. Other fish and shellfish that are tainted with mercury, but in lower amounts, include sea bass, marlin, halibut, pike, walleye, white croaker, largemouth bass, and oysters from the Gulf of Mexico. A pregnant woman who consumes mercury via contaminated fish can pass it on to her fetus through the placenta, with the potential of damaging the brain of the fetus. This can lead later on to learning disabilities, the delay of the mental development of the child, and other neurological problems.

Safe Fish that is Lowest in Mercury

- Blue crab (mid-Atlantic)
- Croaker
- Fish Sticks
- Flounder (summer)
- Haddock Trout (farmed)
- Salmon (wild Pacific)
- Shrimp

Source: The Environmental Working Group (EWG)

High-Fructose Corn Syrup

High-fructose corn syrup (HFCS) is made by changing the sugar glucose in cornstarch into another sugar, fructose. The end product is a combination of fructose and glucose. HFCS is used to extend the shelf-life of processed foods, and it is cheaper than sugar. HFCS is an ingredient that is widely used in many sodas, fruit-flavored drinks, and other processed foods.

According to the April 2004 issue of the *American Journal of Clinical Nutrition*, between 1970 and 1990, the consumption of HFCS in the United States increased by more than 1,000 percent. HFCS now accounts for more than 40 percent of calorie-containing sweeteners that are added to foods and beverages and is the only calorie-containing sweetener used in soft drinks in the United States.

Critics of HFCS say that it contributes to weight gain, tricks the body into wanting to eat more, and causes triglycerides to increase, which is an indicator of risk for cardiovascular disease. Many top health experts think that it is a dangerous chemical concoction.

Protecting Yourself from Food Poisoning

- Clean food thoroughly.
- Drink only pasteurized milk.
- Don't eat raw eggs (cookie dough).
- Cook chicken and pork thoroughly.
- When shopping, choose meat and poultry last, and don't put them in the trunk. The trunk temperature is too hot and bacteria will grow rapidly.
- Don't let meat sit out for longer than one hour during warm weather. If meat sits out too long, bacteria can produce toxins that can cause illness and stay active even during cooking.
- Refrigerate meat and poultry immediately upon arriving home.
- Purchase ground meat or poultry no more than a day or two before you plan to grill it. Otherwise, freeze them. Grill larger cuts of meat, such as steaks, within four days of purchase or freeze them.
- Completely thaw meat and poultry in the refrigerator or just prior to cooking in a microwave.
- Frozen foods do not grill evenly and may be unsafe. Never defrost on the counter—bacteria will begin to grow. It takes about 24 hours to thaw 5 pounds of meat in the refrigerator.

- Clean up juice spills immediately so a raw product does not get on a cooked product. Juice spills should be cleaned with a paper towel. If using a dishcloth to wipe up raw meat or poultry juices, wash it in hot soapy water before using it again.

- Marinate meat and poultry in the refrigerator. Sauce can be brushed on these foods while cooking, but never use the same sauce after cooking that has touched the raw product.

- Unwashed hands are a prime cause of food-borne illness. Whenever possible, wash your hands with hot, soapy water for 20 seconds before handling food. When eating away from home, pack disposable wipes.

- Cook ground beef patties until brown in the middle and juices are clearish with no pink in them when you cut into the meat (160° F). A hamburger can be brown in the middle and still be undercooked.

- The most accurate way to determine doneness is with an instant-read thermometer.

- Though the USDA recommends ground meats should be heated to 160° F to kill microorganisms, the temperature for a steak can be 145° F for "medium rare." A "medium" steak is cooked to 160° F and a "well done" steak is cooked to 170° F.

- Use a tongs or spatula to turn steaks rather than a fork, which punctures the meat and introduces surface bacteria into the interior of the meat.

- Whole poultry should be cooked to 180° F in the thigh. Breast meat should be cooked to 170° F. When poultry is done cooking, juices will run clear with no pink when you cut into the meat.

- If you're preparing steaks, ground meat, and/or poultry at the same time, use a different knife, utensil, or thermometer to check for doneness. For example, don't use the same thermometer to test steaks as you used for hamburgers. Remember to wash thermometers in hot soapy water and rinse in hot water before and after use.

- Discard any food left out for more than two hours or one hour if the temperature is above 90° F. *When in doubt, throw it out!*

Danger Zone: Between 40° F and 140° F.

Irradiation

Irradiation is the exposure of food to ionizing radiation for the purposes of disinfecting, sanitizing, sterilizing, and preserving it, or to eliminate the infestation of insects from food. Irradiation was approved in 2002 in the United States as a treatment for all pests in a small percentage of imported fruits and vegetables. In 2006, irradiation was approved for a wider range of food products, including an expanded number of fruits and vegetables, herbs and spices, wheat flour, white potatoes, pork, and poultry.

There is no government requirement that irradiated foods be labeled as such.

Irradiated food is bombarded with levels of radiation that are 5,000 to 1 million times greater than the level of radiation of a typical chest X-ray.

Many scientists are raising concerns about the possible effects of irradiated foods, which they suspect might destroy vital nutrients and vitamins, as well as alter the chemical structure of the foods. The health risks and long-term effects on human health of irradiated foods is as yet unknown.

The nonprofit public-interest group Public Citizen objects to the irradiation of foods. The group has stated that lab animals that ate irradiated foods developed serious health problems, including the following:

- Premature death
- Fatal internal bleeding

- A rare form of cancer
- High rate of stillbirth and other reproductive problems
- Mutations and other genetic damage
- Organ malfunctioning
- Stunted growth
- Vitamin deficiencies

GMOs

Genetic engineering is the process of modifying the genetic makeup of a live organism. In genetic engineering, scientists take genetic material from one organism and insert it into the permanent genetic code of another organism. Using this process, biotechnologists actually create new forms of organisms. Some examples of genetic engineering include tomatoes that have been altered to slow the softening process, strawberries that have been changed so that they are preserved better after freezing, potatoes that produce toxins to repel or kill pests, and soybeans that can tolerate chemical herbicides. Currently, approximately 40 percent of the corn and 80 percent of the soybeans grown in the United States are genetically engineered. Some health experts warn that foods produced by genetic engineering are hazardous to human health, and some environmental scientists are concerned that genetic engineering might upset the normal balance of ecosystems and the natural order of living things.

In more than 60 countries around the world, GMOs are considered unsafe—including Australia, Japan, and all of the countries in the European Union. In the U.S., the corporation that created them makes so much profit and releases its own studies touting their safety. Unfortunately, they do not even require a label in the U.S.

The affects of these unnaturally altered food products on human health and on the environment are largely unknown. The most common effect observed so far has been allergic reactions to the proteins added to genetically engineered foods in people who are not normally allergic to those particular foods.

To avoid GMOs, avoid these high-risk crops unless labeled organic, non GMO.

- Soy
- Sugar Beets
- Alfalfa
- Canola
- Corn
- Cotton
- Papaya
- Zucchini and Yellow Summer Squash
- Animal products (milk, meat, eggs) because of contamination in feed.

Food Miles, Resources, and the Environment

As a result of globalization and industrialization, the world's food supplies today are grown and processed in fewer locations than ever, which means the food must travel farther to reach consumers' homes. Although highly centralized food production is considered to be efficient and is certainly profitable for large agricultural businesses, many people believe it is harmful to the environment, to consumers, and to rural communities.

Food miles are the distance that a food product travels from its source to the consumer's home. An estimated 80 percent of the energy used in the U.S. food system is consumed by the processing, packaging, transporting, storing, and preparing of food. About 40 percent of the fruit consumed in the United States is produced overseas; a typical fruit or vegetable that is purchased at a grocery store has traveled about 1,500 food miles.

What You Can Do

Buying food that is grown or produced locally significantly reduces food miles and therefore transportation costs, which conserves energy. Locally grown products are fresher, taste better, and are packed with more nutrition, which benefits consumers. Because these foods do not have to travel far, farmers can choose to grow varieties of foods based on flavor rather than on their ability to withstand long journeys to different markets. Knowing who is growing your food can be a powerful thing, and purchasing products from local farmers and food producers keeps more money in your community.

As a consumer, remember to also buy rBGH-free milk, cheese, yogurt, butter, ice cream, infant formula, and meat. Try to buy organic foods as well as local foods.

Organic food is food that is produced by farmers who are committed to the use of renewable resources and the conservation of soil and water to preserve the quality of the environment for future generations. Organic meat, poultry, eggs, and dairy products come from animals that are raised without being given antibiotics or growth hormones. Organic produce is grown without the use of most conventional pesticides, without fertilizers made with synthetic ingredients or sewage sludge, without genetic engineering, and without irradiation. Before a food product can be labeled "organic," a person who is approved by the government inspects the farm where the food is grown to make sure that the farmer is following all the rules required to meet the USDA's organic standards.

"Natural" food is not the same as "organic" food. "Natural" can refer to one or more ingredients that are derived from a plant or animal and added for flavor, not nutrition. For example, mint ice cream's "natural" flavor might refer to the mint that is added to the ice cream.

Guide to Organic Food Terms

When you buy organic foods, look for the "USDA Organic" label. Only foods in the categories "100% organic" and "organic" are permitted to display the USDA Organic Seal. In addition to the other requirements mentioned earlier, organic farmers must practice certain soil and water conservation methods and adhere to rules regarding the humane treatment of animals. The following terms related to organic foods are approved by the USDA:

- **100% organic:** a product that is composed of a single ingredient, such as a fruit, vegetable, meat, milk, and cheese (excluding water and salt)
- **Organic:** a product containing multiple ingredients that are 95% to 100% organic
- **Made with organic ingredients:** 70% of the product's ingredients are organic
- **Contains organic ingredients:** a product made up of less than 70% organic ingredients
- **Fair Trade Certified** is a certification that ensures that farms in developing countries provide humane working conditions and reasonable wages for workers. Under this certification, farms must also use sustainable farming methods that protect the environment. This label most often is found on coffee, tea, chocolate, rice, sugar, grapes, and other fruit.
- **Certified Humane** is a certification that ensures that animals have safe, healthful homes on farms and a diet that does not contain antibiotics or hormones. In addition, farmers comply with the

standards for this certification to help prevent damage to land, air, and water. This label most often is found on eggs, beef, chicken, lamb, pork, and turkey.

- **Rainforest Alliance Certified** is a certification that ensures that local cultures are preserved, that farmers treat workers fairly, and that the use of pesticides is minimal, thereby protecting water, soil, and tropical wildlife. This label most often is found on coffee, orange juice, chocolate, and bananas.
- **Free-range** is a label for poultry that means the bird had access to the outdoors. Unfortunately, the time that a bird spends outside is not regulated, so that time could in fact be minimal.

There are 7 billion people on Earth:

- 2 billion+ are lacking in essential vitamins and minerals
- 1.4 billion are overweight or obese
- 870 million are undernourished

Globesity

An average adult needs to consume a minimum of about 2,000 kilocalories a day. In simple terms, a person who takes in more calories than his or her body uses, will gain weight.

Globesity is a blend of the terms *global* and *obesity*. It refers to the current global public-health crisis that is caused by excessive weight gain. **Obesity** is the condition of a disproportionately high amount of excess body fat and is associated with a variety of debilitating and life-threatening disorders. Obesity is a complex condition, one with serious social and psychological dimensions, that today affects virtually all age and socioeconomic groups. Throughout the world, there are more than 1 billion overweight adults, with at least 300 million of them being obese. Rates of obesity have tripled since 1980 in some parts of North America, the United Kingdom, Eastern Europe, the Middle East, the Pacific Islands, Australasia, and China. In South Africa, obesity rates are about equal to those of the United States, with one out of every three men and more than one out of every two adult women being overweight or obese. The epidemic of obesity is not restricted to the most developed countries, however; the rise in rates of obesity is faster in some developing countries than it is in developed countries.

Almost two-thirds of Americans are currently overweight, and approximately 300,000 Americans die every year of complications related to obesity. The problem of obesity is particularly worrisome because it now affects children even more than adults, as it can lead to early onset of type 2 diabetes, which at one time was virtually never seen in children.

Major Factors for Globesity

1. An increase in consumption of high-energy, high-calorie foods
2. An increase in consumption of foods with few nutrients
3. An increase in consumption of high levels of fats and sugars
4. A decrease in levels of physical activity

The "toxic" environment of the modern world in which we live contributes to globesity.

Some of the contributing factors include:

- **Advertising**
- **Misleading food labels**

- **Sedentary lifestyles**
- **Automated equipment**
- **Prolonged computer use and watching of television**
- **Foods that lack nutrition are available everywhere and nearly anytime:** A large variety of high-fat, high-sugar foods is widely available. These foods taste good and cost less than more healthful foods. There are strips of fast-food restaurants along America's highways and roads and rows of candy at the checkout counters of virtually all convenience and grocery stores.
- **Huge serving sizes:** There are many restaurants that serve all-you-can eat buffets, and many fast-food chains offer "value meals" that contain more food for less money.
- **Advertisements:** There is a barrage of advertising on television and in newspapers and magazines for prepackaged foods and fast foods. Colorfully packaged single servings add to the appeal of processed foods.
- **Physical activity has declined in schools and recess time is being cut:** Most Americans get less exercise than ever before, while driving or riding in a car or other transportation more often than walking or riding bikes to even short destinations.

Americans spend $110 billion a year on fatty and sugary fast foods. Nearly every country in the world now has McDonald's and Pizza Hut restaurants, and Coca-Cola and Pepsi products have been distributed worldwide for many years.

The findings of a new study by the Centers for Disease Control and Prevention (CDC) and the Agency for Healthcare Research and Quality indicate that obesity is taking an incredible toll on the healthcare system of the United States. The report found that the annual cost of obesity in the U.S. is an estimated $147 billion. The researchers involved based their analysis on data from 1998 and 2006 medical and health spending surveys. They defined obesity as a person having a body mass index above 30.

The body mass index (BMI) is a measurement of body fat based on height and weight, and it applies to both adult men and women.

BMI = (Weight in pounds ÷ [Height in inches] × [Height in inches]) × 703

BMI Categories:

- **Underweight:** <18.5
- **Normal Weight:** 18.5-24.9
- **Overweight:** 25–29.9
- **Obese:** 30 or greater

Researchers in the study cited above found that the bulk of healthcare spending related to obesity did not go toward treatments such as bariatric surgery, but instead went to treating diseases associated with obesity. They also noted that a significant amount of excess weight is the best predictor of a person's developing diabetes, the treatment of which accounts for approximately $191 billion annually. They concluded that nearly 10 percent of the money spent on medical conditions in this country is going toward diseases related to obesity, including not only diabetes, but also heart disease and arthritis.

Being overweight and obese are known risk factors for the following:

- Diabetes
- Coronary heart disease
- Hypertension

108

- Stroke
- High blood cholesterol
- Gallbladder disease
- Degeneration of cartilage and bone in the joints
- Sleep apnea and other breathing problems
- Cancers, including breast, colorectal, endometrial, and kidney

Obesity is also associated with the following:

- Complications with pregnancy
- Menstrual irregularities
- Excess body and facial hair
- Incontinence
- Psychological disorders such as depression
- Increased surgical risks
- Increased mortality

Solutions to Reducing and Preventing Obesity

Obesity is a disease largely caused by social and environmental factors, and it urgently needs to be addressed throughout the world. We need to develop strategies that will make it easier for people to make healthful choices. Effective weight management for people who are obese or are at risk of developing obesity requires a range of long-term strategies.

Nutritional experts have recommended the following community-based solutions for decreasing the epidemic of obesity:

- Develop supportive environments through public policies that make a wide variety of low-fat, high-fiber foods more available and accessible, and that provide opportunities for different types of physical activity
- Promote healthful behaviors to motivate, encourage, and enable people to lose weight by
  - Eating more fruits, vegetables, and whole grains
  - Exercising moderately every day for at least 30 minutes
  - Reducing the intake of fatty, sugary foods
  - Eating unsaturated oil-based fats instead of trans fats and saturated animal-based fats
- Make physical activities more accessible by building walking paths and biking lanes, as well as more playgrounds that are safe
- Sponsor and fund after-school recreational programs
- Regulate advertising on television that is aimed at children and mandate equal time for pro-nutrition messages
- Remove and ban fast foods and soft drinks from schools
- Redesign school lunch programs to include more healthful food choices
- Subsidize healthful foods to lower the prices of fruits and vegetables

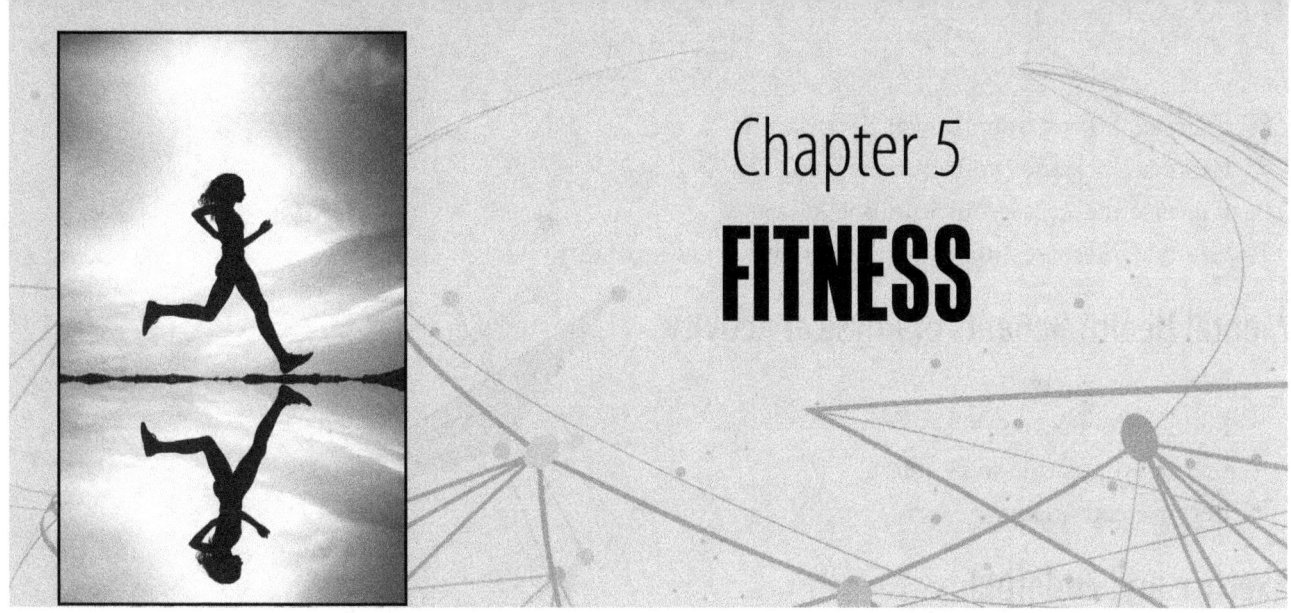

Chapter 5
FITNESS

Physical fitness is not only one of the most important keys to a healthy body, it is the basis of dynamic and creative intellectual activity.

—*John. F. Kennedy*

Regular exercise has many positive benefits—from decreased health risk to weight management to stress reduction. Reflect on some ways that exercise can impact your life.

_____

_____

_____

_____

_____

_____

Why You Should Exercise Regularly?

1. Exercise helps to elevate your mood.
2. Exercise can help you achieve and maintain a healthy weight.
3. Regular exercise will help you sleep better at night.
4. Exercise strengthens your heart and lungs.
5. Being physically active can improve your sex life.
6. Exercise combats chronic diseases.
7. Exercise boosts your energy level.

8. Exercise boosts brain power.
9. Exercise increases your metabolism.
10. Exercise increases your immune system.
11. Exercise increases life expectancy and lowers mortality.

Mental Health Benefits of Physical Activity

- Reduced anxiety
- Reduced depression
- Increased positive self-esteem
- Better sleep quality

Exercise and Endorphins

Many fitness enthusiasts experience something called a "runner's high." You actually don't have to run a marathon to experience this high—moderate exercise releases endorphins which act as powerful hormone-like substances produced in the brain that function as the body's own natural painkillers. During exercise, there is a release of endorphins in the body that are capable of producing feelings of euphoria and a general state of well-being. The feelings produced can be so powerful that they can actually mask pain.

Sedentary Death Syndrome[38]

- Every year in the United States, approximately 300,000 deaths occur due to physical inactivity.
- In the next decade, an expected 2.5 million premature deaths will occur.
- This results in billions of dollars in health-care costs each year.

Characteristics of Sedentary People

- Higher risk of heart attacks
- Higher risk of certain cancers
- Higher risk of hypertension
- Higher risk of osteoporosis
- Greater number of sick days
- Higher stress
- Greater depression and anxiety
- Greater appetite

Inactivity Epidemic[39]

- One in four Americans report no physical activity
- City dwellers versus country folks
- Female versus males
- Higher education versus lower education
- Higher income versus lower income

Children and Inactivity

- Less active
- Higher rates of obesity
- Decreased physical education classes
- Increased diabetes, hypertension, risk of heart disease
- Lower academic performance

College Students

Do you exercise? Why or why not?

_____

_____

_____

_____

_____

*List some reasons why college students do **not** exercise.*

_____

_____

_____

_____

_____

How can we motivate college students to exercise?

_____

_____

_____

_____

_____

Why College Students Exercise—or Don't[40]

Top Exercise Benefits

- Exercise increases my level of physical fitness.
- Exercise improves the way my body looks.
- My muscle tone is improved with exercise.
- Exercise gives me a sense of personal accomplishment.
- Exercise increases my muscle strength.

Top Exercise Barriers

- Exercise tires me.
- Exercise is hard work for me.
- I am fatigued by exercise.
- Exercising takes too much time.
- My family members do not encourage me to exercise.
- No money to join a gym.

Barrier Busters

- Education
- Planning on calendar in ink
- Keeping sneakers in car
- Social support
- Park a few blocks away
- Take stairs
- Take 10-minute walks several times a day
- Hop off the bus/train early and walk
- Turn household chores into calorie burners
- Sign up for a fitness class
- Read schoolwork on stationary bike or stairmaster
- Rewards

Transtheoretical Model (Stages of Change)[41]

James Prochaska and Carlo Diclemente (1982) developed a model of change that is unique in many ways. The model conceptualizes change as entailing a number of stages, which all require alterations in attitude in order to progress. The model depicts change as a cycle as opposed to an all-or-nothing step. The authors contend that it is quite normal for people to require several trips through the stages to make lasting change. Thus, in this sense relapse is viewed as a normal part of the change process as opposed to a complete failure. This does not mean that relapse is desirable or even invariably expected. It simply means that change is difficult, and it is unreasonable to expect everyone to be able to modify a habit perfectly without any slips. The reason the cycle model is so attractive is that it views change as flexible to individual needs. Some people make lasting change quite rapidly; others require a few times through the stages.[42]

Are You Ready to Become More Active?

Precontemplation: No intention to take action within the next six months.

Contemplation: Intends to take action within the next six months.

Preparation: Intends to take action within the next 30 days and has taken some behavioral steps in this direction.

Action: Has changed overt behavior for less than six months.

Maintenance: Has changed overt behavior for more than six months.

Termination: Overt behavior will never return; complete confidence in ability to cope without relapse.

Process of change: Any activity that you initiate to help soothe your thinking, feeling, or behavior.

Nine Major Processes of Change

1. *Consciousness Raising*—Involves providing information regarding the nature and risk of unsafe behaviors and the value and drawbacks of the safer behavioral alternatives.

2. *Dramatic Relief*—Fosters the identification, experiencing, and expression of emotions related to the risk of the safer alternatives in order to work toward adaptive behavior.

3. *Environmental Control*—Allows the individual to reflect on the consequences of his or her behavior for other people. It can include reconsideration of perceptions of social norms and the opinions of people considered important.

4. *Self-Reevaluation*—Entails the reappraisal of one's problem and the kind of person one is able to be, given the problem.

5. *Commitment*—Encourages the person to consider his or her confidence in the ability to change and his or her commitment to doing so.

6. *Social Liberation*—Seeking to help others with similar situations.

7. *Helping Relationships*—Assist the person in a variety of ways, including providing emotional support, modeling a set of moral beliefs, and serving as a sounding board.

8. *Rewards*—Developing internal and external rewards and making them readily but contingently available to improve the probability of the new behavior occurring or continuing.

9. *Countering*—Weighing the pros and cons of the behavior change. The challenge is to tip the balance in favor of making positive changes.

Describe what stage of change you are currently in.

_____

_____

_____

_____

_____

_____

Definitions of Physical Fitness

Physical fitness: Ability to respond to routine physical demands with enough reserve energy to cope with a sudden change.

Aerobic: Oxygen taken into the body is greater than amount of oxygen used by the body.

Examples of aerobic activity:

- Walking
- Jogging/running
- Cycling
- Skiing
- Dancing
- Skating
- Swimming
- Rowing
- Stair climber

Which aerobic activity do you currently perform or would like to start for this semester?

_____

_____

_____

_____

_____

Cardiorespiratory endurance: The ability of the body's circulatory and respiratory systems to supply fuel during sustained physical activity.

Endorphins: Mood-elevating, pain-killing chemicals produced by the brain.

Healthy Benefits of Aerobic Exercise[43]

- Reduction in body weight
- Reduction in blood pressure
- Reduction of low-density lipoprotein (LDL) and total cholesterol
- Increase in high-density lipoprotein (HDL) cholesterol
- Increased insulin sensitivity
- Larger coronary arteries
- Increased heart size
- Increased pumping action
- Increases stamina
- Reduces number of sick days
- Decreases risk of cancer

- Decreases risk of diabetes
- Decreases arthritis symptoms

Anaerobic: High-intensity activity that does not require oxygen to produce the desired energy to carry out the activity. Systems that create energy for activities that last less than five minutes or have frequent rest periods.

Examples of anaerobic activity:

- Sprinting
- Weight lifting

Muscle strength: Force within muscles; measured by the absolute maximum weight you can lift, push, or press.

Muscle endurance: Repeated muscular effort; measured by counting how many times you lift, push, or press a given weight.

Flexibility: Range of motion around specific joints.

Body composition: Relative amounts of fat and lean tissue in body.

- *Body mass index (BMI)*—over 25 is overweight; over 30 is obesity.
- *Waist size*—men with waists larger than 40 inches and women with waists larger than 35 inches are at greatest risk of heart disease.
- *Waist-to-hip ratio (WHR)*—greater than 1 for men or 85 for women is associated with greater risk.
- *Skinfold fat measurement*—a caliper is used to measure the amount of skinfold. Ideal body fat percentages for men are from 7 to 24 percent and for women from 16 to 31 percent.
- *Bioelectrical impedence analysis (BIA)*—noninvasive method; electrical current applied to the body. Based on the theory that lean tissue, which contains large amounts of water and electrolytes, is a good electrical conductor. Fat is a poor conductor.
- *Hydrostatic (underwater) weighing*—gold standard; involves suspending a person attached to a scale in water. Calculated from the relationship of normal body weight to underwater weight.
- *Dual-energy x-ray absorptiometry (DXA)*—x-rays used to quantify the skeletal and soft tissue components of body mass.
- *The Bod Pod*—large fiberglass chamber uses the relationship between pressure and volume to derive body volume.

Check Your Health Status Before Starting an Exercise Program

The American Heart Association and the American College of Sports Medicine (ACSM) recommend that you see a doctor before exercising if:[44]

- you have a heart condition.
- you take medicine for your heart and/or blood pressure.
- you get pains in your chest, left side of your neck, or your left shoulder or arm when you exercise.
- your chest has been hurting for about a month.
- you tend to get dizzy, lose consciousness.
- mild exertion leaves you breathless.
- you are overweight or obese.
- you have diabetes.
- you are over 50 years for women and over 40 for men.

Essential Components of an Exercise Program (FITT)

- *Frequency*—number of sessions per day and week
- *Intensity*—relative physiological difficulty of exercise; risk higher with intensity
- *Type* of exercise based on goals
- *Time*—length of session; inversely related with intensity and compliance

How Much Exercise Is Enough?[45]

The ACSM and the U.S. Surgeon General recommend a minimum of 30 to 60 minutes of moderate activity most days of the week to reduce the risk of cardiovascular disease.

- Aerobics 3–5 times/week; 20–60 minutes; 60–85 percent intensity
- Strength 2–3 times/week; 8–12 repetitions; 2–3 sets per muscle group
- Flexibility 2–3 times/week; especially on the days of strength training

Phases of Exercise Session

1. Warm-up: 5–10 minutes
2. Stretching: 5–10 minutes
3. Workout
4. Cool-down: 5–10 minutes
5. Stretch: 5 minutes

Why Warm Up?

- Prepares your body for physical activity by gradually increasing muscle temperature and metabolism
- Increases blood flow and oxygen delivery to the muscles, protects tendons, and lengthens short, tight muscles
- Gives the body a chance to redirect blood to active muscles
- Gives the heart time to adapt to increased demands
- Stretches the major joints with range-of-motion movements

Why Cool Down?

- Light, gradual movements and stretching to end your physical activity constitute a cool-down.
- Cool-down helps to avoid the pooling of blood in the muscles and to remove metabolic end-products such as lactic acid and carbon dioxide.
- Cool-down reduces muscle soreness, cramps, and stiffness.
- Stretching at the end improves flexibility and prevents injury.

Long-Term Plan of an Exercise Program

1. Beginning (4–6 weeks)—Start slow and with low intensity.
2. Progression (16–20 weeks)—Gradually increase the duration and intensity.
3. Maintenance (lifelong)—Once you've reached the stage of exercising for an hour every day, vary your intensity and duration.

Principles of a Successful Workout

- *Overload*—Placing a greater-than-normal amount of stress on the body in order to make it function at a higher capacity, therefore increasing endurance and/or strength.
- *Specificity*—The type of physical changes you desire in your body relate directly to the type of exercise you choose.
- *Progression*—By gradually increasing the frequency, intensity, and duration of exercise, the body is able to gain improvement in strength and endurance.
- *Intensity*—
  1. *Sedentary* individuals should work toward performing a minimum of 30 minutes of daily moderate activity to decrease risk of cardiovascular disease.
  2. *Moderate* intensity—activities that use energy three to six times the resting metabolic rate (RMR) (40–60 percent max).
  3. *Vigorous*—activities more than six times the RMR (60 percent max).

Heart Rate

- Total number of times the heart contracts per minute; normal rate is 60–80 bpm.
- The quicker your heart recovers after exercise, the better your physical health.
- Use radial or carotid artery for measurement.
- Resting heart rate is most accurately measured upon awakening in the morning.

Estimate Your Maximum Heart Rate[46]

- Take 220 – age = _____ (this is your maximum); standard deviation for this equation is 10–12 beats per minute. 220-18= 202
- Determine your lower-limit exercise heart rate by multiplying your maximum heart rate by 0.6 (60 percent intensity). 202·0.6= 121.2
- Determine your upper-limit exercise rate heart by multiplying your maximum heart rate by 0.8 (80 percent intensity). 202·0.8= 161.8

Your exercise heart rate range is between your upper and lower limits.

For most people, exercising at the lower end of the exercise heart rate range for a longer time is better than exercising at the higher end of the range for a shorter time. Exercising at the lower intensity will improve your overall fitness.

Medications for high blood pressure may affect your heart rate during exercise.

Target Heart Rate (Fat-Burning Zone)

220 – AGE = _____

_____ × .60 = _____ low end of target zone

_____ × .80 = _____ high end of target zone

- Use 60 to 85 percent of your heart rate (HR).
- For weight loss, use 60 to 70 percent of max HR.
- For aerobic conditioning, use 70 to 80 percent of HR.
- If you exercise at higher intensity, it can place a burden on the heart.
- If you don't exercise hard enough, weight loss is impeded.

Target Heart Rate Formula for Women

In a recent study from Northwestern University of nearly 5,500 healthy women, scientists discovered that a decades-old formula for calculating heart rate is largely inaccurate for women, resulting in a number that is too high.

The new formula is:

> **206 − (0.88 × age) = _____ estimated max heart rate.**

The typical goal is to stay within 65 to 85 percent of the estimated maximum heart rate.

The body burns a higher percentage of calories from fat in the 'fat burning zone' or at lower intensities. But, at higher intensities, you burn a greater number of overall calories which is what you should be concerned about when trying to lose weight.

Checking Your Heart Rate

To find your heart rate during exercise, slow down enough to take a fifteen second pulse check. You can find your pulse either on the neck or on the inside of your wrist. Then remember to multiply your pulse by 4, because 15 seconds × 4 = 60 sec (bpm).

You can also purchase a heart monitor to measure your heart rate as you exercise.

Many people are warned to stay within their 'fat burning' zone for the best results, but do you really burn more fat if you 0work at lower intensities?

- We burn more calories from fat at lower intensities of cardio, but we actually burn more total calories from fat and more overall calories at higher intensities, done for shorter time intervals.

Will walking help me lose weight?

- Use a pedometer and count your steps. Step counting is a great way to keep active, aiming to increase your steps by 2,000 per day towards a goal of 10,000 steps per day.

- Walking at 2 mph (3.21 kph), a relatively slow pace, burns about 26 calories per 10 minutes. In 30 minutes the average person burns about 79 calories. Picking up the pace and walking about 3 mph (4.82 kph) almost doubles the benefits of a half hour walk. One burns about 125 calories in a thirty-minute period. As one gets more comfortable walking at slower paces, one can begin to burn even more calories by including a few minutes of extra fast walking or jogging to increase heart rate. When one can walk a mile (1.6 km) in 15 minutes, one burns about 370 calories in an hour.

Other Cardiovascular Measurements

- *MET*—1 MET is the amount of oxygen your body takes in when you're not moving.
- MET values tell you how much harder you're working when compared with rest.

So, exercise performed at 3 METs requires three times the oxygen consumed at rest.

- *WATT*—a measure of power; $\dfrac{\text{force} \times \text{distance}}{\text{time}}$

- *Rate of perceived exertion (RPE)*—A person's own perception of the intensity of his or her exercise can be an accurate gauge of exercise intensity. Multiplying the RPE roughly by 10 approximates the heart rate during exercise. Most people should exercise at an RPE between 3 and 6.

BORG RPE Scale[47]

0. No exertion at all
1. Extremely light
2. Very light
3. Moderate
4. _____
5. Strong (heavy)
6. _____
7. Very strong
8. _____
9. _____
10. Extremely strong

You should always be able to catch your breath and speak comfortably while exercising. Feeling effort or slight discomfort is normal during some exercise. However, you should never sense pain.

Physical Activity Calorie Use Chart[48]

The following chart shows the approximate calories spent per hour by a 100-, 150- and 200-pound person doing a particular activity.

Activity	100 lb	150 lb	200 lb
Bicycling, 6 mph	160	240	312
Bicycling, 12 mph	270	410	534
Jogging, 7 mph	610	920	1,230
Jumping rope	500	750	1,000
Running, 5.5 mph	440	660	962
Running, 10 mph	850	1,280	1,664
Swimming, 25 yds/min	185	275	358
Swimming, 50 yds/min	325	500	650
Tennis singles	265	400	535
Walking, 2 mph	160	240	312
Walking, 3 mph	210	320	416
Walking, 4.5 mph	295	440	572

Major Cardiovascular Training Methods

1. Continuous Training Aerobics

Walking, jogging, swimming, aerobics, cycling, intensity 50 to 85 percent.

- *Long, slow distance workouts (LSD)*—increase the number of red blood cells, hemoglobin concentration, muscle capillaries, mitochondrial volume, and aerobic enzymes.
- LSD workouts enhance your muscles' ability to conserve carbohydrates and rely on fat as fuel, so you become a better fat-burning machine.

2. High-Intensity Interval Training (HIIT)

A very high-intensity effort (85 to 100 percent) designed to enhance competitive performance in a specific sport. The best way to lose fat and increase metabolism.

- Involves periods of max or near-max effort followed by short periods of rest. As intensity increases, the contribution from fat is decreased and the contribution from carbohydrate is increased.
- When you exercise at intensity above your lactate threshold, you burn only carbohydrates.
- Short, intense intervals recruit fast-twitch muscle fibers and complement your strength training by adding muscle definition and size.
- Short, intense workouts increase your anaerobic power and capacity by calling on anaerobic metabolic pathways that don't use oxygen.
- Example of short, intense interval-run, cycle, or row at slightly less than all-out pace for 20 seconds to 60 seconds. Takes one to six minutes to recover. Repeat each cycle five to eight times.
- Long aerobic intervals increase the rate at which you consume oxygen by increasing the volume of blood your heart pumps with each beat *(stroke volume)* and the volume of blood your heart pumps each minute *(cardiac output)*.
- Example of long aerobic intervals: run, cycle, or row for two to five minutes at 90 to 95 percent max heart rate, with recovery of two to five minutes. Repeat each cycle three to five times.

3. Circuit Training Methods

Circuit strength training: This workout is a great calorie-burner and perfect for people who want to get more done in a short period of time and burn more fat! Circuit training could be seen as a form of interval training—high-intensity anaerobic bouts of weight training exercises with low-intensity aerobic recovery periods.

The circuit training is comprised of 6 to 10 strength exercises that are completed one exercise after another. Each exercise is performed for a specified number of repetitions or for a set time before moving on to the next exercise. The exercises within each circuit are separated by a short rest period, and each circuit is separated by a longer rest period.

Some sample circuit workouts include:

- Weight circuit—bench press, leg extension, lat pull-down, hamstring curl, bicep curl, squats, tricep extension, and calf raises
- Core circuit—sit-ups, machine crunches, medicine ball, machine back extension, side twists, leg raises, stability ball, flat floor back lifts, and crunches
- Plyometric circuit—jumping jacks, leg kicks, step-ups, jump up into a squat.

124

4. Circuit Training

Takes the client through aerobic and strength exercises (4–10 stations).

- Each station should be set at 50 to 70 percent of client's functional capacity.

Strength Training Benefits

- Enables muscles to work better
- Capillaries (tiny blood vessels) increase by 50 percent
- Burns fat
- Increases bone density and helps prevent osteoporosis
- Speeds up metabolism and digestion
- Better manage stress and anxiety
- Improves self-esteem
- Improves posture and back pain
- Improves balance

Strength training (and core training): Strength training includes free weights, weight training, plyometrics (jumping jacks, resistance bands), push-ups, sit-ups, and core (torso) exercises. To build muscle, the emphasis should be on higher weight and lower repetitions (6–8) and 3–4 sets. To get cut or look lean, the emphasis should be on lower weight amounts with higher repetitions (8–20), and 2 or 3 sets of several different exercises not lasting more than an hour in total is a general guideline.

In addition, core, or trunk, exercises are some of the most overlooked but most essential supplementary exercises. Core exercises are designed to strengthen your abdomen, your back, and other stabilizer muscles (hip flexors and glutes).

Isometric exercises: Also known as static strength training, this involves muscular actions in which the length of the muscle does not change and there is no visible movement at the joint. Isometric exercises can raise blood pressure significantly for the duration of the exercise. While it will return to a resting level soon after, this can be dangerous for people with hypertension or any form of cardiovascular disease.

Examples of full body isometric exercise:

Plank Bridge

1. Start by lying face down on the ground. Place your elbows and forearms underneath your chest.
2. Prop yourself up to form a bridge using your toes and forearms.
3. Maintain a flat back and do not allow your hips to sag towards the ground.
4. Hold for 10–30 seconds or until you can no longer maintain a flat bridge. Repeat 2–3 times.

Hundred Breaths Exercise

1. Lie face up on a mat with arms by your sides. Bend legs to 90 degrees. Lift your head and shoulders off mat and take 5 short, consecutive inhales, followed by 5 short, consecutive exhales.
2. At the same time, lift arms off mat and pulse them in unison with the breath—palms face up on inhale and down on exhale.
3. Repeat 10 times for a total of 100 breaths.

What Is Your Body Type?

In the 1940s, Dr. William H. Sheldon introduced the theory of Somatypes. His theory described three basic human body types: the endomorph, characterized by a preponderance of bodyfat; the mesomorph, marked by a well-developed musculature; and the ectomorph, distinguished by a lack of either much fat or muscle tissue. He also stated that most people were a mixture of these types.

Ectomorph:
- fragile, thin
- flat chest
- delicate build
- young appearance
- tall
- lightly muscled
- stoop-shouldered
- large brain
- has trouble gaining weight
- muscle growth takes longer

Ectomorphs should concentrate on gaining weight in the form of good lean muscle tissue. Strength training should be fairly heavy and workout pace slower (longer rest periods between sets). Diet should be high in calories (**good quality food, not junk**) and you should eat more frequent meals 5–6 times/day. Aerobic activities should be kept to a minimum, at least until you are happy with your weight gain.

Mesomorph:
- athletic
- hard, muscular body
- overly mature appearance
- rectangular shaped (hourglass shaped for women)
- thick skin
- upright posture
- gains or loses weight easily
- grows muscle quickly

A mesomorph has a naturally fit body, but to maintain it or improve it they should strength-train more often and for longer sessions. You should train with moderate to heavy weights at a moderate pace. If you start getting too bulky, just do lighter weights, more repetitions. A healthy low-fat, higher protein diet will keep you lean and muscular.

Endomorph:
- soft body
- flabby
- underdeveloped muscles
- round shaped
- overdeveloped digestive system
- trouble losing weight
- generally gains muscle easily

An endomorph's biggest concern should be losing the excess body fat. Strength training should be done to get a better muscle-to-fat ratio and to boost metabolism. Endomorphs should eat frequent, small meals—paying attention to the overall calories. Sugars, sweets, and junk food should be eliminated from your diet. Engage daily in some cardio activity.

Working with Weights

Pick calisthenics, free weights, or machine if you intend to work with weights. Just be sure that your strength training includes exercises for every major muscle group, including the muscles of the arms, chest, back, stomach, hips, and legs.

Start with a weight that is comfortable to handle and keep it up for eight repetitions. Gradually add more repetitions until you can complete 12 repetitions. For greater strength conditioning, add more weight and/or more repetitions, in sets of 8 to 12, when the exercise becomes easy.

- *Repetition*—the single performance of an exercise.
- *Set*—a set number of repetitions of the same movement.
- Start with major muscle groups first.
- Maintain proper breathing; exhale on exertion.
- Wait 48 to 96 hours between training the same body part.
- Speed four seconds up, four seconds down.
- To build muscle → decrease reps and increase resistance.
- To tone muscle → increase reps and decrease resistance.
- Change the exercise you perform for each muscle group every four to eight weeks.
- Increase the weight by no more than 10 percent per week.

Why do you need to lift weights in order to lose weight?

- Muscle burns more calories—up to 50 extra calories per pound each day.

Training Frequency[49]

- Beginning: Train entire body two to three days per week.
- Intermediate: Train entire body two to three days per week.
- Split workout: Train each muscle group (upper and lower body) one to two days per week.
- Advanced: Train four to six days per week.
- Elite bodybuilding: Train twice each day for four to five days per week.

Primary Muscle Groups

- Deltoids (shoulders)
- Pectorals (chest)
- Triceps and biceps (back and front of upper arm)
- Quadriceps and hamstrings (front and back of thighs)
- Gluteus maximus (buttocks)
- Trapezius and rhomboids (back)
- Abdomen

Periodization

Instead of doing the same routine month after month, you should change your training program at regular intervals to keep your body working harder while still giving it adequate rest.

For example, you can alter your strength-training program by adjusting the following variables:

- The number of repetitions per set, or number of sets of each exercise
- The amount of resistance used
- The rest period between sets, exercises, or training sessions
- The order of the exercises, or the type of exercises
- The speed at which you complete each exercise

Proper Free Weight-Lifting Techniques

- Warm up before lifting.
- Start slowly and progress gradually.
- Keep weights as close to your body as possible.
- Do most of the lifting with your legs.
- Keep your hips and buttocks tucked in.
- Keep your hands dry or wear gloves.
- Wrap your thumbs around the bar when gripping it.
- When picking up a weight from the ground, keep your back straight and your head level up.
- Use spotters.
- Lower the weights with control.
- Perform all lifts through full range of motion.
- Do not lock the knees or elbows.
- Exhale when exerting the greatest force.
- If you feel pain, stop immediately.
- Stretch and cool down.

Risks of Training

- Overtraining
- Exercise-bulimia
- Injury
- Toxic air
- Congenital defects (hypertrophic cardiomyopathy in athletes)

Signs of Overtraining

- Persistent muscle soreness
- Frequent injuries

- Unintended weight loss
- Nervousness
- Inability to relax
- Lower immunity

RICES Concept for Treatment of Injury:
R   Rest
I   Ice application
C   Compression
E   Elevation
S   Support and stabilization

Benefits of Flexibility Training[50]

- Prevention of injuries
- Relief of muscle strain
- Relaxation
- Relief of soreness
- Improved posture
- Better athletic performance
- Improves coordination and balance
- Improves circulation

Factors That Influence Flexibility[51]

- Muscle temperature—Warm muscles stretch more easily than cold muscles.
- Physical activity—Sedentary individuals are less flexible.
- Injury—Injury can limit range of motion; a good rehab program is advised.
- Body composition—Fat can limit movement and flexibility.
- Age—Flexibility declines with advanced age.
- Disease—Arthritis can make stretching painful.

When Performing Any Stretch

- Do a brief warm-up before stretching.
- Start each stretch slowly, exhaling as you gently stretch the muscle.
- Try to hold each stretch for at least 10 to 30 seconds.
- Stretch all the major muscle groups.
- Repeat the stretch four times.
- Stretch *at least* two to three times per week.

Avoid These Stretching Mistakes

- Don't bounce a stretch. Holding a stretch is more effective and there is less risk of injury.
- Don't stretch a muscle that is not warmed up.
- Don't strain or push a muscle too far. If a stretch hurts, ease up.
- Don't hold your breath.
- Do not stretch a swollen joint.

Ways to Improve Posture[52]

- Sit correctly—distribute weight evenly on both hips, do not cross the legs, keep shoulders back and back straight.
- Stand correctly—hold head up, shoulders back, chest forward, stomach tucked in.
- Lift correctly—keep back straight and bend at knees and hips, keep feet wide, lift object using the leg muscles, not the back.
- Lie in bed correctly—lie on your side with your hips and knees slightly bent; put a flat pillow between your knees.

Temperature Extremes

Exercise in Hot, Humid Weather

- Work out in the cooler part of the day.
- Wear light, porous clothing.
- Slow down and shorten your exercise session.
- Drink 12 to 20 ounces of fluid 15 to 30 minutes before exercising and 6 to 8 ounces every 15 minutes during exercise.

Exercise in Cold Weather

- Dress in layers.
- Protect exposed areas.
- Cover your mouth with a mask or scarf on very cold days.
- Wear special cold-weather clothing.
- Drink plenty of fluids.

Safety

- Do not exercise if you are sick.
- Drink plenty of water—remember that thirst is a sign of dehydration.
- Drink 7 to 10 ounces of water for every 10 to 20 minutes of activity.[53]
- Do not exercise if you are sleep deprived.
- Do not exercise if you are fasting.
- Wear the proper clothing and shoes to prevent injuries.

Physical Activity at Home[54]

- Do housework yourself instead of hiring someone else to do it.
- Work in the garden or mow the grass. Using a riding mower doesn't count! Rake leaves, prune, dig, and pick up trash.
- Go out for a short walk before breakfast, after dinner, or both! Start with 5 to 10 minutes and work up to 30 minutes.
- Walk or bike to the corner store instead of driving.
- When walking, pick up the pace from leisurely to brisk. Choose a hilly route. When watching TV, sit up instead of lying on the sofa. Better yet, spend a few minutes pedaling on your stationary bicycle while watching TV. Throw away your video remote control. Instead of asking someone to bring you a drink, get up off the couch and get it yourself.
- Stand up while talking on the telephone.
- Walk the dog.
- Park farther away at the shopping mall and walk the extra distance. Wear your walking shoes and sneak in an extra lap or two around the mall.
- Stretch to reach items in high places and squat or bend to look at items at floor level.
- Keep exercise equipment repaired and in good condition, and use it!

Stay Motivated

- Develop and exercise good habits.
- Reserve a time slot each day for working out.
- Seek support from family and friends.
- Plan ahead and follow your plan.
- Team up with an exercise buddy or consider hiring a personal trainer.
- Set realistic exercise goals.
- Keep an exercise log and make it visible.
- Have fun with your exercise.
- Add variety.
- Affirm your dedication every day.
- Listen to your body.
- Complement exercise with good nutrition.

If You Relapse: How to Get Back on Track

- Look upon every relapse as a learning experience.
- Stop the negative self-talk—*remember that more than half the people who start an exercise program drop out within the first six months.*
- Reevaluate your goals.
- Start performing some kind of exercise *today*.
- Reevaluate your plan.

Thinking of quitting? Make a list of the benefits of sticking to your exercise program and the risks of quitting. Weigh the pros and cons.

_____

_____

_____

_____

_____

_____

_____

_____

When your life gets more hectic, it gets harder to find time to exercise. How can you incorporate exercise into your daily routine so that it's doable? List all the possible exercise "substitutes" you can count on during your busiest times.

_____

_____

_____

_____

_____

_____

_____

_____

_____

Performance-Boosting Drugs

Androstenodione (Andro-DHEA)

- Androstenodione is a testosterone precursor normally produced by the adrenal glands and gonads.

Claims

- Improves testosterone concentration, increases muscular strength and mass, helps reduce body fat, enhances mood, and improves sexual performance

Risks

- Breast enlargement, increased risk of cardiovascular disease and pancreatic cancer in men, acne, male pattern baldness, and a decrease in "good" (HDL) cholesterol
- In women, high testosterone levels can cause increased body hair, deepening of the voice, and other male characteristics

Anabolic Steroids

- An anabolic steroid is a synthetic derivative of the male hormone testosterone that promotes the growth of the skeletal muscle and increases lean body mass.

Claims

- Enhances performance and improves physical appearance
- Reported to increase lean muscle mass, strength, and the ability to train longer and harder

Risks

- Liver tumors, jaundice, fluid retention, high blood pressure, severe acne, aggression, and other psychiatric side effects
- Men: Shrinking testicles, reduced sperm count, infertility, baldness, and development of breasts
- Women: growth of facial hair, changes in or cessation of the menstrual cycle, enlargement of the clitoris, and deepened voice

Creatine

- Creatine is an amino acid made by the body and stored predominantly in skeletal muscle. Creatine serves as a reservoir to replenish adenosine triphosphate (ATP), a substance involved in energy production.

Claims

- Creatine supplements increase muscle stores of the compound, which theoretically allows athletes to work out harder and longer.

Risks

- Water retention, weight gain, muscle cramping, diarrhea, dehydration, electrolyte imbalances, and kidney dysfunction
- No benefit for lower-intensity, longer-duration exercises

Other Drugs

- *Testosterone*—same side effects as steroids.
- *Human growth hormone (HGH)*—used for muscle growth but causes gigantism—abnormal enlargement of joints, jaw, and skull.
- *Amphetamines*—stimulate central nervous system and delay fatigue but can cause chest pains, increases in blood pressure, and addiction.
- *Caffeine*—increases motor activity and delays fatigue but can cause irritability, abnormal heart rhythm, and insomnia.
- *Erythropoetin (EPO)*—increases red blood cells and the ability to transport oxygen to muscles. Side effects include thickened blood, strokes, and heart problems.

Nutrition for an Active Life

Timing of Meals

- You can exercise three to four hours after a large meal.
- You can exercise one to two hours after a small meal.
- Best preexercise foods: high carbs, low fat, low protein.
- Best postexercise foods: high protein, high carbs.

Preworkout

- A few hours before exercise, choose easily digestible low-fat foods with a little protein, which will give you energy to sustain the exercise and keep your blood sugar from dropping.
- Yogurt and fruit; a peanut butter sandwich; cereal and lowfat milk; egg and toast

Postworkout

- About 15–60 minutes after exercise, eat a recovery snack or meal with plenty of fluids and carbohydrates to refuel, and some protein to rebuild muscle.
- Tuna sandwich; grilled chicken and baked potato; whole wheat pasta and turkey meatballs; protein shake or bar

Fluids

- Consume at least 2 cups of fluid 2 hours before exercising and again 15–20 minutes before exercise.
- If the climate is hot and humid, consume 4 to 6 ounces of water or sports drink every 15 minutes.
- After exercise, consume at least 2 cups per pound of body weight lost during the activity.

Sports Drinks[55]

Activities lasting longer than one hour can leave your body wanting more than just water. Sports drinks, which typically contain about 50 to 70 calories per serving, plus vitamins and minerals, are an easy answer to both the fluid and carbohydrate drain that comes from prolonged activity.

You should be able to complete your 30-minute run or 45-minute step class without the aid of additional carbohydrates, especially if your goal is weight loss. How you choose to refuel during a workout depends on your body's reaction to what you put in it. For sessions lasting less than an hour, water is sufficient so long as you consume at least 4 to 10 ounces every 15 minutes.

Energy Gels and Bars

Energy gels are a relatively new alternative to traditional sports drinks or bars. They feel similar in texture to pudding and are easy to eat and easy for your stomach to digest. They typically contain about 70 to 100 calories and may also include caffeine and other ergogenic aids.

Energy bars are eaten more often as a snack than as an energy replacement during exercise. Today, the market is saturated with numerous flavors and types, each with a different ratio of fats, carbohydrates, and protein.

At 110 to 350 (or more) calories each, energy bars also provide extra vitamins, minerals, and fiber, which ups their nutritional value considerably. But eating an energy gel or bar is not enough. You must consume enough fluid to replace what's been lost as well as to help speed digestion.

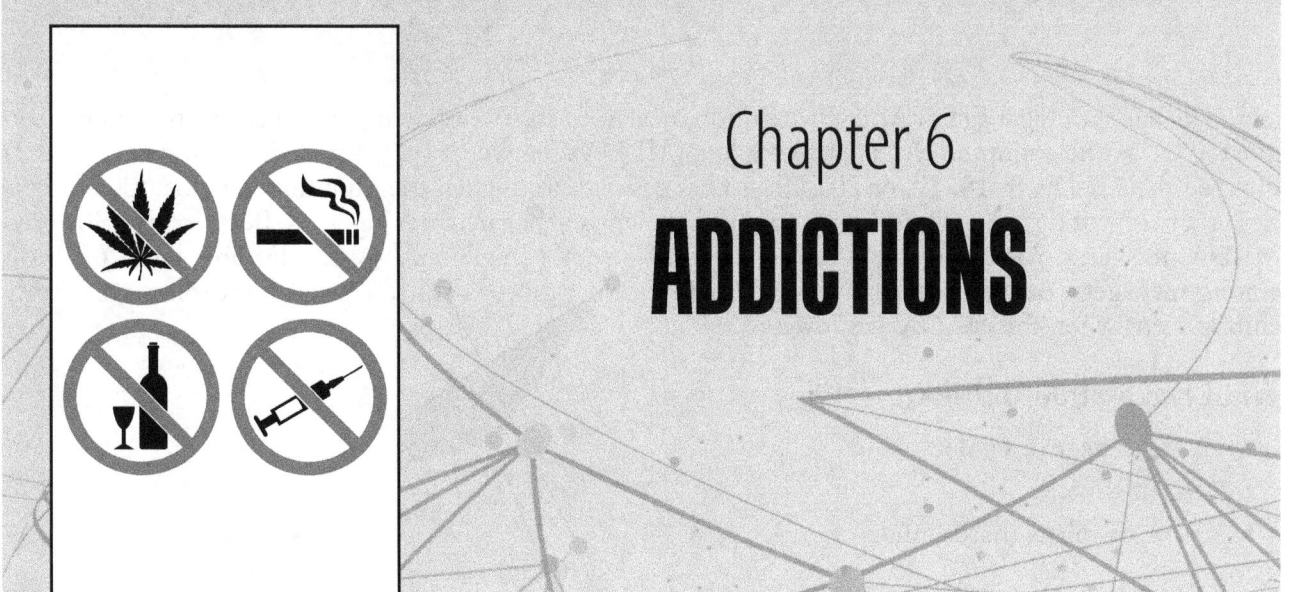

Chapter 6
ADDICTIONS

Alcohol

The use and abuse of alcohol is a serious problem in U.S. society. Alcoholism, also known as alcohol dependence, is a disease that includes four symptoms:

- Craving: A strong need, or compulsion, to drink.
- Loss of control: The inability to limit one's drinking on any given occasion.
- Physical dependence: Withdrawal symptoms, such as nausea, sweating, shakiness, and anxiety, occur when alcohol use is stopped after a period of heavy drinking.
- Tolerance: The need to drink greater amounts of alcohol in order to "get high."

Alcoholism and drug addiction is taking a toll on the American family. As a result, 8.3 million children in the United States, approximately 11 percent, live with at least one parent who is in need of treatment for alcohol or drug dependency. One in four children under the age of 18 are living in a home where alcoholism or alcohol abuse is a fact of daily life. Countless others are exposed to illegal drug use in their families.[119]

Children of addiction are at significantly greater risk for:

- Mental illness or emotional problems, such as depression or anxiety
- Physical health problems
- Learning problems, including difficulty with cognitive and verbal skills, conceptual reasoning, and abstract thinking
- Children whose parents abuse alcohol or drugs are almost three times more likely to be verbally, physically, or sexually abused and four times more likely than other children to be neglected.
- Developing alcoholism or other drug problems[120]

Brief History of Minimum Legal Drinking Age

The Eighteenth Amendment to the U.S. Constitution was passed in 1919 and was made effective in 1920. This started the period known as Prohibition. The Eighteenth Amendment declared that alcohol could not be manufactured, sold, imported, exported, or transported in the United States. In 1933, the Twenty-First Amendment to the Constitution was passed, which repealed the Eighteenth Amendment and made alcohol legal again. After Prohibition, nearly all states restricting youth access to alcohol designated 21 as the minimum legal drinking age (MLDA). Between 1970 and 1975, however, 29 states lowered the MLDA to 18, 19, or 20. These changes occurred when the minimum age for other activities, such as voting, also were being lowered. Scientists began studying the effects of the lowered MLDA, focusing particularly on the incidence of motor vehicle crashes, the leading cause of death among teenagers. Several studies in the 1970s found that motor vehicle crashes increased significantly among teens when the MLDA was lowered.[121]

What Is a Standard Drink?

- 12 oz. of beer or cooler
- 5 oz. of wine
- 1.5 oz. of spirits (hard liquor)

Blood Alcohol Concentration

The amount of alcohol in your body is commonly measured by the blood alcohol concentration (BAC). BAC is the amount of alcohol in the bloodstream. It is measured in percentages. For instance, having a BAC of 0.10 percent means that a person has 1 part alcohol per 1,000 parts blood in the body. BAC is estimated from breath ethanol content measured with a machine commonly referred to as a breathalyzer. BAC can be measured by breath, blood, or urine tests.

The legal intoxication level in most states is 0.08 percent BAC. But because alcohol depresses the central nervous system, causing slowed reactions, one's ability to drive is affected long before a BAC of 0.08 percent is reached.

In some states, drivers under 21 are considered legally impaired at lower levels (perhaps 0.02) as part of a zero-tolerance policy.

Factors Affecting BAC

- *How much* alcohol you drink.
- *How fast you drink.* The quicker you drink, the higher your peak BAC will be. The liver gets rid of alcohol at the average rate of one drink per hour (12 oz. beer, 5 oz. wine, 1 shot of distilled liquor). If a person drinks faster than this, the remainder will circulate in the bloodstream until the liver can get rid of it.
- *Weight.* Heavier people will be less affected by the same amount of alcohol than lighter people. They have more blood and water in their bodies in which to dilute the alcohol.
- *Food in the stomach.* When there is food in the stomach, alcohol is absorbed slower into the bloodstream. The BAC rises more rapidly in those who drink on an empty stomach, because there is no food in which to dilute the alcohol.
- *The type of alcohol you drink.* The stronger a drink is (the higher the alcohol concentration, distilled alcohol first, wine second, beer third), the more quickly it is absorbed. This partially explains why hard liquor has more of an apparent "kick" than wine or beer.
- *Type of mixer used.* Water and fruit juices mixed with alcohol slow the absorption process, whereas carbonated beverages will speed it up. Carbon dioxide speeds the alcohol through the stomach and intestine into the bloodstream, creating a rapid rise in BAC.
- *Temperature of the drink.* Warm alcohol is absorbed quicker than cold alcohol.
- *Drinking history/tolerance.* If there is a long history of drinking, increasing amounts of alcohol are needed to result in the physical and behavioral reactions formerly produced at lesser concentrations.

142

- *General state of emotional and mental health.* Many people seem more susceptible to the effects of alcohol when they are extremely fatigued, have recently been ill, or are under emotional stress and strain. The usual amount of alcohol may result in uncomfortable effects.
- *Other drugs.* Prescription, over-the-counter, illicit, and unrecognized drugs all have potential reactions with alcohol. One should be aware of the additive and synergistic effects when these drugs are mixed with alcohol.
- Males and females respond differently to the effects of alcohol.

Females Process Alcohol Differently than Males

1. *Less body water in women.* For a male and female of the same weight, females have less amount of water in their body. In addition, females tend to weigh less than men. With less of their body containing water and weighing less in general, the same amount of alcohol will be more intoxicating for a female.
2. *Alcohol metabolism.* Females burn up alcohol less rapidly than males. The enzyme (alcohol dehydrogenase) in the stomach that burns up (metabolizes) alcohol is 25 percent less active in females. That means higher levels of alcohol reach their blood and brain, producing greater intoxication.
3. *Hormone levels.* Changing hormonal levels at certain times during the menstrual cycle increase the level of alcohol in a female's body. A woman drinking the same amount of alcohol every day will have twice or more the level of alcohol in her blood during the middle of the menstrual cycle around the time of ovulation as she will at other times in her cycle.

Effects of Alcohol

- *Brain.* Alcohol is a "downer." It directly affects the brain cells. Unclear thinking, staggering, and slurred speech may result. Drinking a high concentration of alcohol in a short period of time can suppress the centers of the brain that control breathing, causing a person to pass out or even die.
- *Eyes.* Alcohol causes blurred vision.
- *Heart.* Alcohol can increase the workload of the heart. Irregular heartbeat and high blood pressure can result. At intoxicating doses, alcohol can decrease heart rate, lower blood pressure and respiration rate, and result in decreased reflex responses and slower reaction times.
- *Liver.* Alcohol can poison the liver. Prolonged use causes extensive damage and organ failure.
- *Stomach/Pancreas.* Alcohol irritates the digestive system. Vomiting and ulcers may result.
- *Kidneys.* Alcohol can stop the kidneys from maintaining a proper balance of body fluids and minerals.
- *Veins/Arteries.* Alcohol widens blood vessels, causing headaches and loss of body heat. It also lowers body temperature—this dilation of vessels actually causes heat loss from the extremities, which makes you more vulnerable to the cold. The vessels constrict in the first place to conserve heat, a defense the alcohol undoes.
- *Blood.* Alcohol reduces your body's ability to produce blood cells, resulting in anemia and/or infections.
- *Muscles.* Alcohol can cause muscle weakness, including weakness of the heart muscle.

Path of Alcohol in the Body

1. *Mouth:* alcohol enters the body.
2. *Stomach:* some alcohol gets into the bloodstream in the stomach, but most goes on to the small intestine.
3. *Small intestine:* alcohol enters the bloodstream through the walls of the small intestine.

4. *Heart:* pumps alcohol throughout the body.
5. *Brain:* alcohol reaches the brain.
6. *Liver:* alcohol is oxidized by the liver at a rate of about 0.5 oz. per hour. Alcohol is converted into water, carbon dioxide, and energy.

Results of Chronic Alcohol Abuse

- Cirrhosis of the liver
- Damage the frontal lobes of the brain
- Overall reduction in brain size and increase in the size of the ventricles (fluid-filled cavities)
- Alcoholism (addiction to alcohol) and tolerance to the effects of alcohol and variety of health problems
- Vitamin deficiency—because the digestion system of alcoholics is unable to absorb vitamin B_1 (thiamine), a syndrome known as *Wernicke's encephalopathy* may develop. This syndrome is characterized by impaired memory, confusion, and lack of coordination.
- Further deficiencies of thiamine can lead to *Korsakoff's syndrome*. This disorder is characterized by amnesia, apathy, and disorientation.

Fetal Alcohol Syndrome (FAS)

Compared to normal babies, babies born with FAS have:

- Smaller heads and brains
- Some degree of mental retardation
- Poor coordination
- Hyperactivity
- Abnormal facial features
- Lower IQ

Positive Effects of Alcohol

- In light drinkers, there is less heart disease than in nondrinkers. However, there's more cancer.
- Recommendation: one drink a day for women and two drinks a day for men.
- Wine has the healthiest effects.

Binge Drinking

Binge drinking is defined as drinking five or more drinks on the same occasion (i.e., within a few hours) on at least 1 day in the past 30 days.

Consequences

Drinking by college students aged 18 to 24 contributes to an estimated 1,700 student deaths, 599,000 injuries, and 97,000 cases of sexual assault or date rape each year.[123]

What Happens to Your Body When You Get Alcohol Poisoning?

- Alcohol depresses nerves that control involuntary actions such as breathing and the gag reflex (which prevents choking). A fatal dose of alcohol will eventually stop these functions. Alcohol has a built-in safety feature: We either vomit or pass out before we have a chance to kill ourselves. The trick is not to do the two things simultaneously; otherwise you risk choking on your own vomit.
- When people pass out, their bodies continue to absorb alcohol. The amount of alcohol in the blood can reach dangerous levels, and they can die in their sleep. Continue to check on someone who has gone to sleep drunk. Do not leave that person alone.
- A person's BAC can continue to rise even while he or she is passed out. Even after a person stops drinking, alcohol in the stomach and intestine continues to enter the bloodstream and circulate throughout the body. It is dangerous to assume the person will be fine by sleeping it off.

Critical Signs for Alcohol Poisoning

- Mental confusion, stupor, coma, or person cannot be roused
- Vomiting
- Seizures
- Slow breathing (fewer than eight breaths per minute)
- Irregular breathing (10 seconds or more between breaths)
- Hypothermia (low body temperature), bluish skin color, paleness

What Should I Do If I Suspect Someone Has Alcohol Poisoning?

- Know the danger signals.
- Do not wait for all symptoms to be present.
- Be aware that a person who has passed out may die.
- If there is any suspicion of an alcohol overdose, call 911 for help. Don't try to guess the level of drunkenness.

What Can Happen to Someone with Alcohol Poisoning That Goes Untreated?

- Victim may choke on his or her own vomit.
- Breathing may slow, become irregular, or stop.
- Heart may beat irregularly or stop.
- Hypothermia (low body temperature) may result.
- Hypoglycemia (too little blood sugar) may lead to seizures.
- Untreated severe dehydration from vomiting can cause seizures, permanent brain damage, or death.
- Even if the victim lives, an alcohol overdose can lead to irreversible brain damage.

Reasons to Quit Binge Drinking

- To reduce chances of dying in a car crash
- To decrease the chance of falls or other injuries
- To do better in school
- To decrease chances of being date raped
- To prevent blackouts
- To decrease the chance of contracting STDs

- To save money
- To feel better
- To have more energy
- To be nicer to my friends
- To reduce my weight
- To reduce the number of headaches
- To reduce stomach pain
- To reduce risk of developing an addiction to alcohol
- To decrease chance of developing medical problems related to drinking

Advertising and Youth

- Greater exposure to alcohol advertising contributes to an increase in drinking among underage youth. Specifically, for each additional ad a young person saw above the average for youth, he or she was 1 percent more likely to drink. For each additional dollar spent per capita on alcohol advertising in a local market, young people drank 3 percent more.
- Young people view approximately 20,000 commercials each year, of which nearly 2,000 are for beer and wine. For every "just say no" or "know when to say when" public service announcement, teens will view 25 to 50 beer and wine commercials.[125]

Alcohol Marketing and the African American Community[128]

- Alcohol is the drug most widely used by African American youth.[129]
- Although African American youth drink less than other youth, there is evidence from public health research that, as they age, African Americans suffer more from alcohol-related diseases than other groups in the population.[130]
- References to alcohol were more frequent in rap (47 percent of songs had alcohol references) than other genres such as country-western (13 percent), top 40 (12 percent), alternative rock (10 percent), and heavy metal (4 percent); and 48 percent of these rap songs had product placements or mentions of specific alcohol brand names.

Alcohol and Medication Effects

1. *Antibiotics*—Alcohol decreases effects of certain antibiotics.
2. *Anticoagulants (Coumadin)*—Alcohol can lead to risk of life-threatening hemorrhages.
3. *Antidepressants and antipsychotics*—Alcohol increases the sedative effect of some, impairing mental skills required for driving. A chemical called tyramine, found in some beers and wine, interacts with some antidepressants, such as monoamine oxidase inhibitors, to produce a dangerous rise in blood pressure.
4. *Aspirin* (nonnarcotic pain relievers)—Some of these drugs cause stomach bleeding and inhibit blood from clotting; alcohol can exacerbate these effects.
5. *Acetaminophen*—liver damage.
6. *Antihistamines*—Alcohol may intensify the sedation.
7. *Narcotic pain relievers*—The combination of opiates and alcohol enhances the sedative effect of both substances, increasing the risk of death from overdose.

8. *Sedatives and hypnotics* (sleeping pills) cause severe drowsiness in the presence of alcohol.
9. *Antidiabetic medication*—Alcohol causes blood sugar fluctuations.
10. *Antiseizure medications*—Alcohol increases the risk of drug-related side effects.
11. *Antiulcer medications* increase the availability of a low dose of alcohol under some circumstances.
12. *Cardiovascular medications*—Alcohol causes dizziness, fainting.

Withdrawal

People who drink all the time build up a tolerance to alcohol. Symptoms are:

- Tremors
- Irritability
- Anxiety
- Heightened sensitivity to light, noise, and pain
- Hallucinations
- Convulsions

Hangovers

- *Coffee or a cold shower will not sober you up if you're drunk.*
- Only time can make you sober. It takes approximately two hours for each ounce of alcohol to work its way out of your bloodstream.
- Drink plenty of water.
- Do not take Tylenol or other medications.

How Can You Tell If a Friend Has a Drinking Problem?

If your friend has one or more of the following warning signs, he or she may have a problem with alcohol:

- Getting drunk on a regular basis
- Lying about how much alcohol he or she is using
- Believing that alcohol is necessary to have fun
- Having frequent hangovers
- Feeling run-down, depressed, or even suicidal
- Having "blackouts"—forgetting what he or she did while drinking

Cigarettes

Smoking is the most preventable cause of premature death in our society.

Who Smokes?[131]

According to the Centers for Disease Control and Prevention (CDC), 44.5 million U.S. adults were current smokers in 2004 (the most recent year for which numbers are available). This is 20.9 percent of all adults (23.4 percent of men, 18.5 percent of women)—more than one out of five people.

When broken down by race/ethnicity, the numbers for 2004 are as follows:

American Indians/Alaska Natives	33.4 percent
Whites	22.2 percent
African Americans	20.2 percent
Hispanics	15.0 percent
Asian Americans	11.3 percent

Health Effects of Smoking

- About half of all Americans who continue to smoke will die because of the habit.
- Nearly one of every five deaths is related to smoking. Cigarettes kill more Americans than alcohol, car accidents, suicide, AIDS, homicide, and illegal drugs combined.
- Smoking is the number-one preventable cause of death.
- About 87 percent of lung cancer deaths are caused by smoking.

Diseases Caused by Long-Term Smoking

- Cancer of the lung, mouth, nose, voice box, lip, tongue, nasal sinus, esophagus, throat, pancreas, bone marrow (myeloid leukaemia), kidney, cervix, liver, bladder, and stomach
- Lung diseases such as chronic obstructive pulmonary disease, which includes chronic bronchitis and emphysema
- Coronary artery disease, heart disease, heart attack, and stroke
- Ulcers of the digestive system
- Osteoporosis and hip fracture
- Poor blood circulation in feet and hands, which can lead to pain and, in severe cases, gangrene and amputation

The Female Body

When calling attention to public health problems, we must not misuse the word 'epidemic.' But there is no better word to describe the 600-percent increase since 1950 in women's death rates for lung cancer, a disease primarily caused by cigarette smoking. Clearly, smoking-related disease among women is a full-blown epidemic.

—David Satcher, MD, PhD

148

- Women who smoke greatly increase their risk of heart disease (the leading killer among women) and stroke.
- Some studies suggest that smoking cigarettes dramatically increases the risk of heart disease among younger women who are also taking birth control pills.

The specific effects of tobacco smoke on the female body include:

- reduced fertility.
- menstrual cycle irregularities or absence of menstruation.
- menopause reached one or two years earlier.
- increased risk of cancer of the cervix.
- greatly increased risk of stroke and heart attack if the smoker is over age 35 years and taking a oral contraceptive pill.

Birth control and smoking increases risk of:

- blood clots
- strokes
- heart disease

The Male Body

The specific effects of tobacco smoke on the male body include:

- lower sperm count
- higher percentage of deformed sperm
- reduced sperm mobility
- changed levels of male sex hormones
- impotence, which may be due to the effects of smoking on blood flow and damage to the blood vessels of the penis.

The Effects of Maternal Smoking

- Increased risk of miscarriage, stillbirth, and premature birth
- Low birth weight, which may have a lasting effect on the growth and development of children. Low birth weight is associated with an increased risk for early puberty, and in adulthood an increased risk for heart disease, stroke, high blood pressure, and diabetes.
- Increased risk of cleft palate and cleft lip
- Paternal smoking can also harm the fetus if the nonsmoking mother is exposed to passive smoking
- If the mother continues to smoke during her baby's first year of life, the child has an increased risk of ear infections, respiratory illnesses such as pneumonia, croup and bronchitis, sudden infant death syndrome (SIDS), and meningococcal disease.

Ingredients in Tobacco

Cigarettes, cigars, and smokeless and pipe tobacco consist of dried tobacco leaves, as well as ingredients added for flavor and other properties. More than 4,000 individual compounds have been identified in tobacco and tobacco smoke. Among these are more than 60 compounds that are known carcinogens (cancer-causing agents).

Some of the compounds found in tobacco smoke include:

- Tar (burning of tobacco)
- Carbon monoxide
- Cyanide
- Benzene
- Formaldehyde
- Methanol (wood alcohol)
- Acetylene (the fuel used in welding torches)
- Ammonia

How Nicotine Affects the Body

Nicotine is highly addictive. It is both a stimulant and a sedative to the central nervous system. The ingestion of nicotine results in almost immediate pleasure because it causes a discharge of epinephrine from the adrenal cortex. This stimulates the central nervous system and other endocrine glands, which causes a sudden release of glucose. Stimulation is then followed by depression and fatigue, leading the abuser to seek more nicotine. Nicotine is absorbed readily from tobacco smoke in the lungs, and it does not matter whether the tobacco smoke is from cigarettes, cigars, or pipes.

Nicotine is a drug found naturally in tobacco. It is highly addictive, as addictive as heroin and cocaine. The body becomes physically and psychologically dependent on nicotine.

Nicotine also is absorbed readily when tobacco is chewed. With regular use of tobacco, levels of nicotine accumulate in the body during the day and persist overnight. Thus, daily smokers or chewers are exposed to the effects of nicotine for 24 hours each day. Nicotine taken in by cigarette or cigar smoking takes only seconds to reach the brain but has a direct effect on the body for up to 30 minutes.

Research has shown that stress and anxiety affect nicotine tolerance and dependence. Stress hormones reduces the effects of nicotine; therefore, more nicotine must be consumed to achieve the same effect. This increases tolerance to nicotine and leads to increased dependence.

Addiction to nicotine results in withdrawal symptoms when a person tries to stop smoking. For example, a study found that when chronic smokers were deprived of cigarettes for 24 hours, they had increased anger, hostility, and aggression, and loss of social cooperation. Persons suffering from withdrawal also take longer to regain emotional equilibrium following stress. During periods of abstinence and/or craving, smokers have shown impairment across a wide range of psychomotor and cognitive functions, such as language comprehension.[133]

Tobacco companies are required by law to report nicotine levels in cigarettes to the Federal Trade Commission (FTC) but in most states are not required to show the amount of nicotine on the cigarette brand labeling. The actual amount of nicotine available to the smoker in a given brand of cigarettes may be different from the level reported to the FTC. In one regular cigarette, the amount of nicotine ranges between about 1 mg and 2 mg.[134]

Although 70 percent of smokers want to quit and 35 percent attempt to quit each year, fewer than 5 percent succeed. The low rate of successful quitting and the high rate of relapse are due to the effects of nicotine addiction.[135]

Research has found that even smoking as few as one to four cigarettes a day can have serious health consequences, including an increased risk of heart disease and a higher risk of dying at an earlier age.

Secondhand Smoke

Secondhand smoke, also known as environmental tobacco smoke (ETS) or passive smoke, is a mixture of two forms of smoke from burning tobacco products:

- *Sidestream smoke:* smoke that comes from the end of a lighted cigarette, pipe, or cigar.
- *Mainstream smoke:* smoke that is exhaled by a smoker.

Secondhand smoke is classified as a "known human carcinogen." Secondhand tobacco smoke contains over 4,000 chemical compounds. Secondhand smoke can be harmful in many ways.

In the United States alone, secondhand smoke is responsible for:[136]

- an estimated 35,000 to 40,000 deaths from heart disease in people who are not current smokers.
- about 3,000 lung cancer deaths in nonsmoking adults.
- other respiratory problems in nonsmokers, including coughing, phlegm, chest discomfort, and reduced lung function.
- 150,000 to 300,000 lower respiratory tract infections (such as pneumonia and bronchitis) in children younger than 18 months of age, which result in 7,500 to 15,000 hospitalizations.
- increases in the number and severity of asthma attacks from about 200,000 to 1 million asthmatic children.
- increases in the risk of sudden infant death syndrome (SIDS) and middle ear infections in young children.
- low birth weight in babies whose mothers are exposed to ETS.

Third-hand Smoke

Doctors from Mass General Hospital for Children in Boston coined the term "third-hand smoke" to describe chemicals from the cigarettes by-products that cling to smokers' hair and clothing as well as to household fabrics, carpets, and surfaces, even after secondhand smoke has cleared.

This third-hand smoke is NOT cleared, even if you open a window or turn on a fan, and this poses a huge threat to children especially. Third-hand smoke is an invisible, cancer-causing toxic brew of gases and particles. This residue includes heavy metals and even radioactive materials that young children can get on their hands and ingest, especially if they're crawling or playing on the floor.

Spit (Smokeless Tobacco)

- Cancer of the mouth and pharynx
- Leukoplakia (white sores in the mouth that can lead to cancer)
- Gum recession, or peeling back of gums
- Bone loss around the teeth
- Abrasion of teeth
- Bad breath

Clove cigarettes, also called kreteks, are imported mainly from Indonesia and contain 60 to 70 percent tobacco and 30 to 40 percent ground cloves, clove oil, and other additives. The chemicals in cloves have been implicated in cases of asthma and other lung diseases.

Bidis are flavored cigarettes imported mainly from India. They are hand-rolled in an unprocessed tobacco leaf and tied with strings on the ends. Their popularity has grown in recent years in part because they come in a variety of candy-like flavors such as strawberry, vanilla, and grape, they are usually less expensive than regular cigarettes, and they often give the smoker an immediate buzz. They have higher levels of nicotine (the addictive chemical in tobacco) and other harmful substances such as tar and carbon monoxide. And because they are thinner than regular cigarettes, they require about three times as many puffs per cigarette. They are also unfiltered.

Most *cigars* have as much nicotine as several cigarettes. When cigar smokers inhale, nicotine is absorbed as rapidly as it is with cigarettes. For those who do not inhale, it is absorbed more slowly through the lining of the mouth. Smoking cigars causes cancers of the lung, oral cavity (lip, tongue, mouth, throat), larynx (voice box), esophagus, and probably cancers of the bladder and pancreas. Cigar smokers have a greater risk of dying from cancer of the oral cavity, larynx, or esophagus compared with nonsmokers.

Hookah smoking, which started in the Middle East, involves burning flavored tobacco in a water pipe and inhaling the smoke through a long hose. It has recently become popular among young people, especially around college campuses. It is marketed as being a safe alternative to cigarettes because the percent of tobacco in the product smoked is low. *This claim for safety is not true.* The water does not filter out many of the toxins, and hookah smoke contains varying amounts of nicotine, carbon monoxide, and other hazardous substances. Several types of cancer, as well as other health effects, have been linked to hookah smoking.

Are Menthol Cigarettes Safer than Other Brands?

Menthol cigarettes are not safer than other brands and may even be more dangerous. Menthol cigarettes produce a cool sensation in the throat when smoke is inhaled. People who smoke menthol cigarettes can inhale deeper and hold the smoke inside longer than smokers of nonmenthol cigarettes. About one-fourth of all cigarettes sold in the United States are flavored with menthol, and these cigarettes are especially popular among African American smokers.

Benefits of Quitting Smoking

- Smoking cessation has major and immediate health benefits for men and women of all ages. Benefits apply to persons with and without smoking-related disease.
- Former smokers live longer than continuing smokers. For example, persons who quit smoking before age 50 have one-half the risk of dying in the next 15 years compared with continuing smokers.
- Smoking cessation decreases the risk of lung cancer, other cancers, heart attack, stroke, and chronic lung disease.
- Women who stop smoking before pregnancy or during the first three to four months of pregnancy reduce their risk of having a low-birth-weight baby to that of women who never smoked.
- The health benefits of smoking cessation far exceed any risks from the average 5-pound (2.3-kg) weight gain or any adverse psychological effects that may follow quitting.
- The risk of having lung cancer and other smoking-related cancers is related to total lifetime exposure to cigarette smoke, as measured by the number of cigarettes smoked each day, the age at which smoking began, and the number of years a person has smoked.
- People who stop smoking at younger ages experience the greatest health benefits from quitting. Those who quit in their 30s may avoid most of the risk due to tobacco use. However, even smokers who quit after age 50 substantially reduce their risk of dying early. The argument that it is too late to quit smoking because the damage is already done is not true.

Quitting[138]

After 20 minutes: Your blood pressure drops to a level close to that before the last cigarette. The temperature of your hands and feet increases to normal.

152

After 8 hours: The carbon monoxide level in your blood drops to normal.

After 24 hours: Your chance of a heart attack decreases.

Within 3 months: Your circulation improves and your lung function increases up to 30 percent.

In 1 to 9 months: Coughing, sinus congestion, fatigue, and shortness of breath decrease; cilia (tiny hair-like structures that move mucus out of the lungs) regain normal function in the lungs, increasing the ability to handle mucus, clean the lungs, and reduce infection.

After 1 year: The excess risk of coronary heart disease is half that of a smoker's.

After 5 years: Stroke risk is reduced to that of a nonsmoker.

After 10 years: The lung cancer death rate is about half that of a continuing smoker's. The risk of cancer of the mouth, throat, esophagus, bladder, kidney, and pancreas decreases.

After 15 years: The risk of coronary heart disease is that of a nonsmoker's.

Cost of Smoking

How much do you pay for a pack of cigarettes? _____

How many cigarettes are you smoking each day? _____

Cost per day: _____

Cost per week: _____

Cost per month: _____

Cost per year: _____

Total cost to date: _____

What else could I have done with this money?

_____

_____

_____

_____

Drug Addiction

Why do college students use drugs?

_____

_____

_____

_____

Reasons for Drug Use

- Deal with stress
- Experimentation
- Pleasure/boredom
- Peer pressure
- Self-discovery
- Social interaction
- Rebelliousness

Addiction is characterized by compulsive drug craving, seeking, and use that persists even in the face of negative consequences.

All addicting drugs act on a single aspect of the brain: dopamine. Dopamine allows us to experience pleasure. Love, sex, food, movies, alcohol, and drugs all release chemicals in our brain that we feel as pleasure.

Our Brains Get Accustomed to Alcohol and Drugs

Drugs can cause such intense pleasure that we can stop wanting to do anything else but take drugs. Our brains change and get accustomed to having drugs. They stop reacting as strongly to the substance so we need to take more and more. The disease of addiction occurs as permanent changes in our brain develop from the repeated exposure to alcohol or addicting drugs.

Dependency Factors

- Genetic factors inherited from our parents
- Our childhood experiences (both with our family and peer group)
- Our current peer group and life situation
- The level of addictive and risk potential of the drugs we use

Common Dependency Defenses

- *Denial:* Refusing to admit or acknowledge that our drinking or using has become a problem. (I can quit any time I want to. My using isn't that bad.)
- *Isolation:* Removing ourselves from the company of family and friends for the purpose of maintaining a chemical habit.
- *Rationalization:* Giving reasons to explain why we drink or use. (I drink because I hate my job.)
- *Blaming:* Transferring responsibility for our behavior to other people. (I wouldn't drink if my spouse treated me right.)
- *Projection:* Rejecting our own feelings by ascribing them to someone else. (Why is that stupid idiot being so hostile?)
- *Minimizing:* Refusing to admit the magnitude of the amount used. (I only have a couple of drinks. It's not a problem.)

Diagnostic and Statistical Manual—IV (DSM-IV)[139]

The DSM-IV defines dependency as a maladaptive pattern of substance use leading to clinically significant impairment or distress as manifested by three (or more) of the following, occurring at any time in the same 12-month period:

- Substance is often taken in larger amounts or over longer period than intended.
- Persistent desire or unsuccessful efforts to cut down or control substance use.
- A great deal of time is spent in activities necessary to obtain the substance (e.g., visiting multiple doctors or driving long distances), use the substance (e.g., chain smoking), or recover from its effects.
- Important social, occupational, or recreational activities given up or reduced because of substance abuse.
- Continued substance use despite knowledge of having a persistent or recurrent psychological or physical problem that is caused or exacerbated by use of the substance.
- Tolerance, as defined by either:
  1. Pharmacological tolerance—need for real amounts of the substance in order to achieve intoxication or desired effect.
  2. Behavioral tolerance—an individual learns to adjust to the presence of drugs.
  3. Cross-tolerance—tolerance to a particular drug results in tolerance to chemically similar drugs.
  4. Reverse tolerance—markedly diminished effect with continued use of the same amount.
- Withdrawal, as manifested by either characteristic withdrawal syndrome for the substance, or the same (or closely related) substance is taken to relieve or avoid withdrawal symptoms.

Drug Interactions

- *Additive*—the cumulative effects of two or more substances added together.
- *Antagonistic*—drugs that negate each other's effects.
- *Synergism*—combined effects of two drugs are greater than if they were simply added together.

Examples:

- Alcohol and marijuana intensify each other's effects.
- Alcohol and tranquilizers → coma.
- Alcohol and antihistamines → deep sleep.
- Birth control and antibiotics → cancel the potency of the pill.
- Marijuana and cocaine → deadly heart rate and blood pressure.

In contrast to prescription drugs, illegal drugs are not manufactured in controlled environments under strict standards of quality. You never know what quality and quantity you are really getting, or with what cheaper poison an unscrupulous dealer may have diluted the drug.

Some of the side effects of illegal drugs could actually limit your ability to have the "good time" you might have thought the drug was going to provide. The side effects multiply, compound, and can cause permanent damage the more frequently you take the drugs.

Side Effects

- Confusion
- Anxiety
- Paranoia
- Panic attacks
- Nausea
- Shaking
- Headache
- Schizophrenic and psychotic behavior
- Hostile and aggressive behavior
- Violence, often for no apparent reason
- Periods of severe mental and emotional disturbance, and possible permanent mental illness
- Potentially permanent damage to brain, liver, kidneys, and heart

Most Dangerous Over-the-Counter Drugs

- Aspirin
- NSAIDs
- Acetaminophen
- Nasal sprays
- Laxatives
- Eye drops
- Cough syrup

Club Drugs

The term "club drugs" refers to a wide variety of drugs being used by young people at dance clubs, bars, and all-night dance parties ("trances" or "raves"). Because many of these drugs are colorless, tasteless, and odorless, they can be secretly added to beverages by individuals who want to intoxicate or sedate others.

Short-Term Effects

- Stimulation
- Loss of inhibition
- Headache
- Nausea or vomiting
- Slurred speech
- Loss of motor coordination
- Wheezing

Long-Term Effects

- Unconsciousness
- Cramps

- Weight loss
- Muscle weakness
- Depression
- Memory impairment
- Damage to cardiovascular and nervous systems
- Sudden death

Widely Used Club Drugs[142]

Ecstasy[143]

Also known as MDMA (methylenedioxymethamphetamine), Ecstasy is a stimulant that combines the effects of amphetamines and hallucinogens. Street names for MDMA include Ecstasy, Adam, XTC, hug, beans, and love drug. Ecstasy is known to cause brain damage. MDMA also is neurotoxic, and depletes serotonin from the brain.

Side Effects

- Increased heart rate, blood pressure, and body temperature
- Nausea and sweating
- Convulsions
- Hallucinations
- Paranoia
- Severe depression
- Breathing problems

Life-Threatening Effects

- High doses can cause a sharp increase in body temperature (malignant hyperthermia), leading to muscle breakdown and kidney and cardiovascular system failure.
- Can cause hyponatremia and swelling of the brain and overstimulation of the nervous system.

Rohypnol

Known as the "date rape drug," Rohypnol is a central nervous system depressant that produces sedative-hypnotic effects, muscle relaxation, and amnesia. Rohypnol has been a concern for the last few years because of its abuse as a date rape drug. People may unknowingly be given the drug, which, when mixed with alcohol, can incapacitate victims and prevent them from resisting sexual assault. Also, Rohypnol can be lethal when mixed with alcohol and/or other depressants.

Rohypnol produces sedative-hypnotic effects including muscle relaxation and amnesia; it can also produce dependence. Rohypnol is not approved for use in the United States and its importation is banned. Illicit use of Rohypnol began in Europe in the 1970s and started appearing in the United States in the early 1990s, where it became known as "rophies," "roofies," "roach," "rope," and the "date rape" drug.

Another very similar drug is clonazepam, marketed in the United States as Klonopin and in Mexico as Rivotril. It is sometimes abused to enhance the effects of heroin and other opiates.[144]

Ketamine

A rapid-acting general anesthetic and hallucinogen, ketamine produces a wide range of feelings, from weightlessness to out-of-body or near-death experiences. Ketamine (ketamine hydrochloride) is a central nervous system depressant that produces a rapid-acting dissociative effect. It was developed in the

1970s as a medical anesthetic for both humans and animals. Ketamine is often mistaken for cocaine or crystal methamphetamine because of its similar appearance.

Also known as K, Special K, Vitamin K, Kit Kat, Keller, Super Acid, and Super C, ketamine is available in tablet, powder, and liquid form. So powerful is the drug that, when injected, there is a risk of losing motor control before the injection is completed. In powder form, the drug can be snorted or sprinkled on tobacco or marijuana and smoked. The effects of ketamine last from 1 to 6 hours, and it is usually 24 to 48 hours before the user feels completely "normal" again.

GHB (Gamma Hydroxybutyrate)[145]

Originally available over the counter in health food stores to aid bodybuilders, GHB and other synthetic steroids are also used for their euphoric effects. GHB is a central nervous system depressant once used by many bodybuilders and athletes. In the 1980s, GHB was widely available over the counter in health food stores, and bodybuilders used it to lose fat and build muscle. GHB has been given nicknames such as Grievous Bodily Harm, G, Liquid Ecstasy, and Georgia Home Boy.

In 1990, the FDA banned the use of GHB except under the supervision of a physician because of reports of severe side effects, including euphoric and sedative effects similar to the effects experienced after taking Rohypnol (the "date rape" drug.) Because it clears from the body relatively quickly, it is often difficult to detect when patients go to emergency rooms and other treatment facilities.

Amphetamines

Amphetamines refers to various nervous system stimulants. Originally given to World War II soldiers to combat fatigue, amphetamines are widely prescribed for weight control and suppression of appetite. Because amphetamines trigger the release of adrenalin, they produce energy and alertness, and the user feels "wired."

1. Methamphetamine

Methamphetamine is made easily in laboratories with relatively inexpensive over-the-counter ingredients. These factors combine to make methamphetamine a drug with high potential for widespread abuse.

Methamphetamine is commonly known as "speed," "meth," and "chalk." In its smoked form, it is often referred to as "ice," "crystal," "crank," and "glass." It is a white, odorless, bitter-tasting crystalline powder that easily dissolves in water or alcohol. It was used originally in nasal decongestants and bronchial inhalers. Methamphetamine's chemical structure is similar to that of amphetamine, but it has more pronounced effects on the central nervous system. Like amphetamine, it causes increased activity, decreased appetite, and a general sense of well-being. The effects of methamphetamine can last six to eight hours. After the initial "rush," there is typically a state of high agitation that in some individuals can lead to violent behavior.[146]

Methamphetamine releases high levels of the neurotransmitter dopamine, which stimulates brain cells, enhancing mood and body movement. It also appears to have a neurotoxic effect, damaging brain cells that contain dopamine and serotonin. Over time, methamphetamine appears to cause reduced levels of dopamine, which can result in symptoms like those of Parkinson's disease, a severe movement disorder.[147]

Short-Term Effects

- Increased heart rate, blood pressure, and metabolism
- Feelings of exhilaration
- Energy
- Increased mental alertness
- Aggression, violence, psychotic behavior
- Suicidal thoughts.

158

Long-Term Effects

- Memory loss
- Cardiac and neurological damage
- Impaired memory and learning
- Tolerance, addiction
- Respiratory problems
- Irregular heartbeat
- Extreme anorexia
- Hyperthermia and convulsions can result in death.
- Increased heart rate and blood pressure can cause irreversible damage to blood vessels in the brain, producing strokes.
- Its use can result in cardiovascular collapse and death.

  Withdrawal symptoms are very intense. The user crashes intensely and desperately craves the drug.

2. *Ritalin and Adderall*

The United States uses approximately 90 percent of the world's ritalin. Most recently, major civil suits have been brought against Novartis, the manufacturer of ritalin, for fraud in the overpromotion of ADHD and ritalin. Furthermore, their addiction and abuse potential is based on the capacity of these drugs to drastically and permanently change brain chemistry. Studies of amphetamine show that short-term clinical doses produce brain cell death. Similar studies of ritalin show long-lasting and sometimes permanent changes in the biochemistry of the brain.[148]

All stimulants impair growth not only by suppressing appetite but also by disrupting growth hormone production. This poses a threat to every organ of the body, including the brain, during the child's growth. The disruption of neurotransmitter systems adds to this threat.

These drugs also endanger the cardiovascular system and commonly produce many adverse mental effects, including depression.

Side Effects

- Suicidal thoughts
- Nervousness and insomnia
- Hypersensitivity
- Anorexia
- Nausea, dizziness
- Palpitations
- Headache
- Drowsiness
- Blood pressure and pulse changes, both up and down
- Tachycardia, angina, cardiac arrhythmia
- Abdominal pain
- Weight loss
- There have been rare reports of Tourette's syndrome.
- Toxic psychosis has been reported.[149]

Hallucinogens

Hallucinogens are drugs that cause hallucinations—profound distortions in a person's perceptions of reality. Under the influence of hallucinogens, people see images, hear sounds, and feel sensations that seem real but do not exist. Some hallucinogens also produce rapid, intense emotional swings.

Hallucinogens cause their effects by disrupting the interaction of nerve cells and the neurotransmitter serotonin. Distributed throughout the brain and spinal cord, the serotonin system is involved in the control of behavioral, perceptual, and regulatory systems, including mood, hunger, body temperature, sexual behavior, muscle control, and sensory perception.

Short-Term Effects

- Increased heart rate and blood pressure
- Impaired motor function
- Possible decrease in blood pressure and heart rate
- Panic, aggression, and violence

Long-Term Effects

- Memory loss
- Numbness
- Nausea/vomiting
- Loss of appetite
- Depression
    1. **LSD (lysergic acid diethylamide):** This hallucinogen produces unpredictable effects, depending on the amount taken, the surroundings in which the drug is used, and the user's personality, mood, and expectations. LSD is tasteless, odorless, and colorless, and can be taken in different ways (e.g., on a sugar cube or tablet or placed on a blotter and licked). Behavior effects lasts six to eight hours. Fear or panic may lead to a "bad trip." Flashbacks are sometimes experienced because the drug remains in the spinal fluid.
    2. **Peyote:** Used by Aztec Indians for religious rituals. Until 1990 it was legally used in the United States by Native Americans. It comes from a cactus, and is the psychoactive agent in mescaline. Peyote takes effect within 30–90 minutes and stays in the body for about 10 hours. Hallucinogenic effects last for about two hours. Tolerance for peyote forms quickly.
    3. **Psilocybin:** Also called magic mushrooms or "shrooms"; the hallucinations produced by psilocybin are both visual and auditory. Psilocybin can produce responses from uncontrolled laughter to depression. Hallucinogenic effects are experienced within 30 minutes and can last 3 to 8 hours.
    4. **PCP** ("PeaCe Pill"): PCP is an anesthetic capable of producing hallucinations; it can be smoked or ingested. Absorption is rapid and effects are experienced quickly. Acute effects lasts four to six hours. One may be in a state of confusion for 8 to 24 hours. Sometimes marijuana is laced with PCP, called a "killer joint" or "sherms." High doses can lead to coma, death, and violent behavior.

Heroin[150]

Heroin is a highly addictive drug, and its use is a serious problem in America. Recent studies suggest a shift from injecting heroin to snorting or smoking because of increased purity and the misconception that these forms of use will not lead to addiction.

Heroin is processed from morphine, a naturally occurring substance extracted from the seedpod of the Asian poppy plant. Heroin usually appears as a white or brown powder. Street names for heroin include "smack," "H," "skag," and "junk." Other names may refer to types of heroin produced in a specific geographical area, such as "Mexican black tar."

Short-Term Effects

Heroin abuse is associated with serious health conditions, including fatal overdose, spontaneous abortion, collapsed veins, and infectious diseases, including HIV/AIDS and hepatitis. It's one of the most deadliest drugs due to risk of overdose.

Heroin is a depressant. The short-term effects of heroin abuse appear soon after a single dose and disappear in a few hours. After an injection of heroin, the user reports feeling a surge of euphoria ("rush") accompanied by a warm flushing of the skin, a dry mouth, and heavy extremities. Following this initial euphoria, the user goes "on the nod," an alternately wakeful and drowsy state. Mental functioning becomes clouded due to the depression of the central nervous system.

In addition to the effects of the drug itself, street heroin may have additives that do not readily dissolve and result in clogging the blood vessels that lead to the lungs, liver, kidneys, or brain. This can cause infection or even death of small patches of cells in vital organs.

Long-Term Effects[151]

With regular heroin use, tolerance develops. This means the abuser must use more heroin to achieve the same intensity or effect. As higher doses are used over time, physical dependence and addiction develop. Chronic users may develop collapsed veins, infection of the heart lining and valves, abscesses, cellulitis, liver disease, and HIV. Pulmonary complications, including various types of pneumonia, may result from the poor health condition of the abuser, as well as from heroin's depressing effects on respiration.

Withdrawal, which in regular abusers may occur as early as a few hours after the last administration, produces drug craving, restlessness, muscle and bone pain, insomnia, diarrhea and vomiting, cold flashes with goose bumps ("cold turkey"), kicking movements ("kicking the habit"), and other symptoms. Major withdrawal symptoms peak between 48 and 72 hours after the last dose and subside after about a week.

Cocaine[152]

Cocaine is a powerfully addictive stimulant that directly affects the brain. Pure cocaine was first extracted from the leaf of the coca bush, which grows primarily in Peru and Bolivia, in the mid-nineteenth century. In the early 1900s, it became the main stimulant drug used in most of the tonics/elixirs that were developed to treat a wide variety of illnesses. Today, cocaine is a Schedule II drug, meaning that it has high potential for abuse but can be administered by a doctor for legitimate medical uses, such as a local anesthetic for some eye, ear, and throat surgeries.

There are basically two chemical forms of cocaine: the hydrochloride salt and the "freebase." The hydrochloride salt, or powdered form of cocaine, dissolves in water and, when abused, can be taken intravenously (by vein) or intranasally (in the nose). *Freebase* refers to a compound that has not been neutralized by an acid to make the hydrochloride salt. The freebase form of cocaine is smokable. The high from snorting may last 15 to 30 minutes, and that from smoking may last 5 to 10 minutes.

Cocaine is generally sold on the street as a fine, white, crystalline powder, and is also known as "coke," "C," "snow," "flake," or "blow." Street dealers generally dilute it with such inert substances as cornstarch, talcum powder, and/or sugar, or with such active drugs as procaine (a chemically related local anesthetic) or with other stimulants such as amphetamines.

Short-Term Effects

- Increased heart rate, blood pressure, and metabolism
- Feelings of exhilaration
- Energy
- Increased mental alertness
- Increased body temperature

Long-Term Effects[153]

Long-term effects include rapid or irregular heart beat, reduced appetite; weight loss, heart failure, chest pain, respiratory failure, nausea, abdominal pain, strokes, seizures, headaches, and malnutrition.

High doses of cocaine and/or prolonged use can trigger paranoia. When addicted individuals stop using cocaine, they often become depressed. This also may lead to further cocaine use to alleviate depression. Prolonged cocaine snorting can result in ulceration of the mucous membrane of the nose and can damage the nasal septum enough to cause it to collapse. Cocaine-related deaths are often a result of cardiac arrest or seizures followed by respiratory arrest.

When people mix cocaine and alcohol consumption, they are compounding the danger each drug poses and unknowingly forming a complex chemical experiment within their bodies. The human liver combines cocaine and alcohol and manufactures a third substance, cocaethylene, which intensifies cocaine's euphoric effects, while possibly increasing the risk of sudden death.

Crack

Crack is the street name given to the freebase form of cocaine that has been processed from the powdered cocaine hydrochloride form to a smokable substance. The term *crack* refers to the crackling sound heard when the mixture is smoked. Crack cocaine is processed with ammonia or sodium bicarbonate (baking soda) and water, and heated to remove the hydrochloride.

Because crack is smoked, the user experiences a high in less than 10 seconds. This rather immediate and euphoric effect is one of the reasons that crack became enormously popular in the mid-1980s. Another reason is that crack is inexpensive both to produce and buy. Smoking crack cocaine can produce a particularly aggressive paranoid behavior in users.

Inhalants[154]

Inhalants are breathable chemical vapors that produce psychoactive (mind-altering) effects. Although people are exposed to volatile solvents and other inhalants in the home and in the workplace, many do not think of inhalable substances as drugs because most of them were never meant to be used in that way.

Young people are likely to abuse inhalants, in part because inhalants are readily available and inexpensive. Sometimes children unintentionally misuse inhalants that are found in household products.

Short-Term Effects

- Impaired physical coordination
- Facial flushing
- Mental confusion
- Hallucinations
- Asphyxia

Long-Term Effects

- Sudden Sniffing Death
- Blindness
- Fatal damage of liver and kidneys

How to Avoid Tempting Situations

In certain situations, especially if you are having a bad day, you will find that you are tempted to drink, smoke, or take drugs. It is important to figure out ahead of time how to make sure you will not drink when you are tempted. Here are some tips from other students about ways to cope without drinking when life gets you down.

- Think of something pleasant you can do for yourself or for a friend.
- Telephone a sober friend.
- Exercise: go for a walk, play a sport, or go to the gym.
- Take a hot bath or shower.
- Watch a light movie or read a book or magazine.
- Write your feelings down in a notebook.
- Listen to music.
- *Surround yourself with positive people.*

Treatment

Chemical dependency is a treatable condition. The first goal of treatment is abstinence. The chemically dependent person must stop using alcohol or drugs. This sometimes requires a period of medical detoxification.

Once alcohol and/or drug use is stopped, individuals may honestly feel that they have the desire and ability to remain sober. This period can last days, weeks, or months before cravings (the obsessive pressure to use) return. To reduce the risk of a relapse the person must address personal problems and life issues related to the chemical dependency.

Participation in various self-help programs such as **Alcoholics Anonymous** and **Narcotics Anonymous** can help break addictions.

Medicinal Marrijuana

Currently, the two main cannabinoids from the marijuana plant that are of medical interest are THC and CBD.

THC can increase appetite and reduce nausea. THC may also decrease pain, inflammation (swelling and redness), and muscle control problems.

Unlike THC, CBD is a cannabinoid that doesn't make people "high." These drugs aren't popular for recreational use because they aren't intoxicating.

- Medical marijuana is used for
    - pain
    - nausea
    - muscle spasms
    - anxiety
    - multiple sclerosis
    - low appetite

o   sleep problems
o   autism
o   epilepsy (seizure disorders)
o   and other conditions

• The health benefits of medical marijuana include relief from pain and muscle spasm, nausea associated with chemotherapy, and anorexia. The side effects of medical marijuana are minimal when used at low doses and include dry mouth and fatigue. At higher doses, side effects include dizziness, paranoia, and psychoactive effects.

• In states where medical marijuana is legal, shops, often called dispensaries, sell marijuana products in a variety of forms. Medical marijuana is available in edible forms (candies or cookies), oils and extracts, and as the plant that can be smoked or otherwise inhaled. Dispensaries require a medical marijuana card before they will sell products. How people can get a medical marijuana card varies by state. It requires a prescription from a licensed health-care professional.

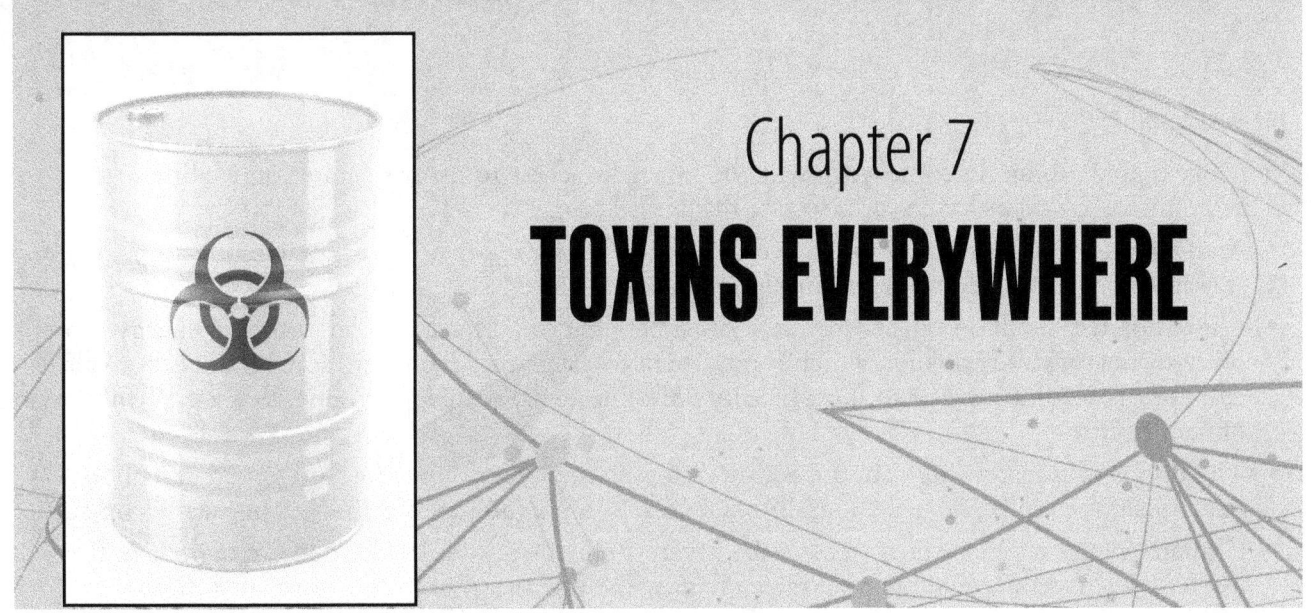

Chapter 7
TOXINS EVERYWHERE

....

We do not inherit the earth from our ancestors; we borrow it from our children.
—*Native American Proverb*

....

As human beings, we are all part of the environment, and the ways in which we interact with our environment greatly influences the quality of our lives. **Environmental health** is all of the physical, chemical, biological, social, and psychosocial factors in the environment. It also refers to the theories and practices involved in assessing, correcting, controlling, and preventing factors in the environment that can potentially adversely affect the health of present and future generations.

Environmental hazards are dangers in the environment. They might be biological, chemical, physical, psychological, or sociological dangers. The exploitation of natural resources, such as the destruction of forests, the building of new land, and the contamination of water have caused alarming changes in the environment in recent decades, often harming the most vulnerable people in the world who depend on natural resources for survival.

The physical environment also has significant impacts on people's health behaviors. Approximately 70 percent of deaths caused by cancer are a result of lifestyle and environmental factors, including the following:

- Being overweight and obese
- Low fruit and vegetable intake
- Lack of physical activity
- Smoking
- Using alcohol in excess
- Unsafe sex
- Urban air pollution

Did you know?

- More than 2.4 billion people worldwide do not have access to proper sanitation facilities, and 1 billion people do not have access to safe drinking water.

- An estimated 2 million children die every year—6,000 a day—from preventable infections that are spread by contaminated water or unsafe sanitation facilities.

- Approximately 2 billion of the world's poorest people do not have regular access to energy supplies for heating and cooking, which forces them to clear trees from rain forests and other valuable forests for firewood or to burn heavily polluting fuels, such as kerosene, that are harmful to human health.

- The disproportionately high energy consumption by the richest countries has caused greenhouse gas emissions to spike, which could ultimately result in potentially dire changes in Earth's climates.

- Climate changes are expected to have the greatest effect on some of the poorest regions in the world. Possible consequences of climate changes include the alteration of rainfall patterns that will impact agriculture, the spreading of diseases such as malaria, and more catastrophic and frequent extreme weather events that the people of poor countries are ill equipped to handle, such as the frequent hurricanes and tsunamis.

Any time that humans change the environment, there potentially will be repercussions related to health, including the risk of increased incidences of diseases. In the book *Collapse: How Societies Choose to Fail or Succeed*, Jared Diamond presents many examples of cultures that died out because they refused to change their traditional habits of how they interacted with the environment. For example, the Rapa Nui, a group of people who lived on a Polynesian island, were obsessed with building large stone figures called moai, which they moved using wooden ramps made from trees. The Rapa Nui eventually clear-cut the entire island, which led to the extinction of animals and plants, starvation, and social chaos.

The consequences of international trade, economic policies, and the control of land by governments or the most powerful have caused immense poverty, hunger, and less access to food among the less powerful. The United States consumes far more energy and raw materials per person than any other country on Earth. The richest 20 percent of people in the highest-income countries account for 86 percent of total expenditures for private consumption worldwide, while the poorest 20 percent of people account for just 1.3 percent.

Some of the major factors that contribute to a worsening of environmental hazards include the growth of urbanization, industrialization, populations, and the production of disposable products and containers.

Many human activities generate wastes and residues as by-products. These by-products include the following:

1. Human body wastes

2. Trash and garbage from food and other packages

3. Organic wastes, such as grass and shrub clippings

4. Construction and manufacturing wastes, such as scrap wood, metal, contaminated water, chemical solvents, heat, and noise

5. Transportation wastes, such as carbon monoxide, nitrous oxides, hydrocarbons, other pollutants, and used motor oil

6. Energy-production wastes, including wastes from mining, electrical power production (combustion of coal), nuclear power plants (whose wastes are radioactive), and the manufacture of weapons

Overpopulation

The health of the environment would not be an issue if there were unlimited land, water, and resources on Earth. However, this is not the case. The human population on Earth continues to grow and is estimated to be greater than 6 billion people, all of whom must share the same piece of the resources pie but with smaller and smaller portions. Overpopulation has created other problems, such as the potential to cause health epidemics; as people meet more and more people, the more and different types of contagious germs and viruses can be picked up and passed along to others. Overpopulation also creates the problems of sanitation and pollution, which can also contribute to health epidemics. However, overpopulation is just one of the factors in the worsening conditions of the environment. Other factors include how and where people choose to live and how they produce, consume, and often waste Earth's resources.

Human Behaviors that Impact the Environment:

- Agricultural burning
- Over-consumption of resources
- Failure to recycle
- Improper disposal of toxic wastes
- Improper disposal of human wastes
- Improper disposal of trash
- Overuse and misuse of pesticides
- Overcrowding
- Depletion of soils by over-farming
- Removal of vegetation
- Urban sprawl
- Over-fishing
- Removal of trees without replanting
- Inefficient use of fuels
- Urbanizing farmland
- Urban growth where water is scarce
- Eating and mass producing meat
- Wars
- Environmental disasters caused by humans

Environmental Disasters that Impact Our Air

9/11 Dust

The destruction of the World Trade Center (WTC) on September 11 of 2001 was the largest environmental disaster that New York City had ever experienced. Amid all the rubble, asbestos was of great concern not only to government agencies in New York City, but also to the public. Asbestos from the destruction of the two towers settled at Ground Zero and in nearby apartments, office buildings, and schools.

Facts about Asbestos:

- It is a fibrous form of mineral silicates.
- Its fibers can lodge in the lungs, abdomen, brain, and heart of humans.
- It can cause mesothelioma, a fatal cancer more painful and devastating even than AIDS.
- It can cause asbestosis, which causes death in humans by cutting off their blood supply.
- It can lay dormant in the lungs for years and then suddenly become active (almost like a ticking time bomb inside the lungs).
- Large but unknown amounts of asbestos are contained within the structures of older commercial and residential buildings.

Fallout from 9/11:

- Some scientists have claimed that the Environmental Protection Agency and other government agencies mislead the public about the asbestos fallout.
- Thousands of workers and visitors were exposed to asbestos and now have the cough characteristic of such exposure.
- Police officers, firefighters, and other first responders became ill with respiratory problems including asthma, cancer (leukemia), and kidney and heart problems. A study released by the Mount Sinai Medical Center in 2004 found that three-fourths of them had contracted diseases.

In the largest health study ever conducted by doctors at Mount Sinai Medical Center, findings indicate that the negative impacts on the health of the thousands of rescue and recovery workers who labored at Ground Zero have been more widespread and persistent than had previously been thought, and that these negative impacts are likely to linger far into the future. An estimated 70 percent of the nearly 10,000 workers who were tested at Mount Sinai between 2002 and 2004 reported that they had newly developed or substantially worsened respiratory problems while or after working at Ground Zero. The study is among the first to show that many respiratory problems, such as sinusitis and asthma, as well as gastrointestinal problems related to these problems that were first reported by those who worked at Ground Zero persisted or worsened in the years after 9/11. The study reported that the toxic nature of the dust resulting from the collapse of the towers would remain a serious health issue in the city for years to come. The dust contained tiny shards of glass, which could become lodged in the lungs, as well as a mixture of toxic and carcinogenic substances, including asbestos and dioxin, that could all have the potential for causing cancer decades into the future.

As the health problems caused by 9/11 continue to expand, concern is also growing about the cost of health care for the responders and workers, especially the 40 percent who either did not have health insurance at the time or who lost the health care coverage provided by their employers after they became too ill to continue working.

Chernobyl

On April 26, 1986, testing was being conducted in a nuclear reactor of the Chernobyl nuclear power plant in Ukraine. The plant was located just 80 miles from Kiev, the capital of Ukraine. Both errors in the design of the reactor and errors in judgment of the personnel working at the nuclear power plant caused the cooling water to boil. This disastrous condition created reactor stress that caused energy production to increase to 10 times the normal level. Temperatures inside the reactor reached more than 2,000° C, causing the fuel rods to melt and the cooling water to continue to boil. The extreme pressures that built up in the cooling water pipes caused them to crack, which, in turn, allowed steam to escape from the power plant.

In the middle of the night, the steam that had escaped caused a massive explosion, blowing the roof off the building, igniting a major fire, and forming a huge toxic cloud in the atmosphere that contained an estimated 185 to 250 million curies of radioactive material. The fire and the explosion instantly killed 31 people. The next day, more than 135,000 people were evacuated from within a 30-kilometer radius of the power plant, an area that the government called the special zone. Because the high levels of radioactivity that had escaped from the nuclear reactor were expected to exist in that area for centuries to come, the evacuation of the special zone was permanent. In the meantime, winds blew the huge radioactive cloud north and northwest, and it soon covered a large portion of Europe—even reaching the Netherlands—causing governments to prohibit consumption of fresh fruits and vegetables.

Many scientists have tried to estimate the number of victims that suffered from symptoms caused by radiation from the Chernobyl accident; however, there is still no reliable data. The WHO reported that about 800,000 people worked to extinguish the, restore the reactor, and clean up pollutants in the first year after the accident. People who had lived in the area near Chernobyl at the time of the accident suffered from a variety of health problems. Immediately after the accident, hundreds of people were diagnosed with radiation sickness. In addition, there was a dramatic increase in the number of cases of thyroid cancer and leukaemia, especially in nearby Belarus. Children suffered from birth defects that caused cancer and heart diseases. The combination of all the health problems related to the Chernobyl accident and the fear of death from radiation caused mental illness in many children, and suicide rates increased by 1,000 percent in the areas nearby.

Three Mile Island

On March 28, 1979, the cooling system of a reactor at the Three Mile Island nuclear power plant near Harrisburg, Pennsylvania, failed. The cooling water drained away from the reactor instead of over it, with the result of a partial meltdown of the reactor core. This caused a release into the atmosphere of approximately one-thousandth the amount of radiation as was released during the Chernobyl explosion.

Studies have indicated that the radiation from the Three Mile Island nuclear reactor contributed to premature deaths, the development of cancers, and birth defects of people who lived in the area at the time of the nuclear meltdown. Dairy farmers also reported that many of their animals had died because of the accident.

Love Canal

By 1920, the Hooker Chemical plant had turned an area in Niagara Falls into a chemical disposal site. A nearby city bought the dumpsite for one dollar with the intention of using it for urban expansion. Blocks of homes and a school were subsequently built, and the neighborhood was named Love Canal.

Children who lived in the neighborhood often became ill, and no one knew why. Residents of Love Canal regularly experienced miscarriages and birth defects. When research was conducted, more than 130 pounds of the highly-toxic carcinogenic TCDD, a form of dioxin, was discovered in Love Canal. In addition, the total of 20,000 tons of waste that was present in the landfill appeared to contain more than 248 different types of chemicals. However, none of the chemicals were removed from the dumpsite. Instead, the dumpsite was sealed, and the surrounding area was cleaned up and declared safe. Today, the Love Canal dumpsite is known as the first and one of the most disastrous human-caused environmental events of the twentieth century.

The Exxon Valdez

In 1989, the oil-tanker ship *Exxon Valdez* spilled more than 30 million gallons of crude oil into Prince William Sound, just off the coast of Alaska. The spill created a huge oil slick that settled on top of the water. Despite intensive cleanup efforts, the oil spill killed an estimated 250,000 seabirds, 2,800 sea otters, 250 bald eagles, and 22 killer whales. Wildlife biologists and medical researchers now know that particular components of the oil, called polycyclic aromatic hydrocarbons, are deadly. These components can work their way through air, water, soil, and food. They can cause reproduction difficulties, genetic damage, central nervous system problems and respiratory problems, and cancer. Exxon Mobil, the owner of the *Exxon Valdez*, paid approximately 3.5 billion dollars in fines and cleanup costs associated with the oil spill.

Newtown Creek

Exxon Mobil is responsible for another environmental disaster, an underground oil spill and leakage into Newtown Creek in New York City. Newtown Creek remains one of the nation's most polluted waterways, affecting the health of people in the city. To date, an estimated 17 million gallons of oil have leaked into the creek. The leakage amounts to approximately 6 million gallons more than was spilled by the *Exxon Valdez* in 1989 and remains the largest underground oil spill in U.S. history.

In Greenpoint, a community in Brooklyn that borders the Newtown Creek, residents complained about strong petroleum odors and experienced the worst of the spill. Neighborhoods in Queens, including Long Island City, West Maspeth, and Sunnyside, also border the creek. Riverkeeper, an environmental advocacy group dedicated to protecting the ecological integrity of the Hudson River, has warned that the Newtown Creek spill and leakage pose a serious threat to the health of the people who live near the banks of the creek in both Queens and Brooklyn.

New York State Attorney General Andrew Cuomo stated, in reference to the spill and the company's record-shattering profits of $39.5 billion in 2006, "Exxon Mobil has proven itself far less than a model corporate citizen, placing its greed for windfall profits over public safety and the well-being of the environment."

The Gulf War

In August of 1990, Iraqi forces invaded Kuwait, igniting the Gulf War and resulting in two major environmental disasters. The first incident was an oil spill about 10 miles off the shore of Kuwait caused by the dumping of oil from several tankers and the opening of the valves of an offshore terminal. The second incident involved the burning of 650 oil wells in Kuwait. An estimated one million tons of crude oil was lost, making this the largest oil spill in history. In the spring of 1991, as many as 500 oil wells were still burning, and the last one was not extinguished until November.

The oil spills of the Gulf War considerably damaged the environment of the Persian Gulf. Within several months of the spills, the tainted water killed 20,000 seabirds and caused serious damage to marine flora and fauna. The fires in the oil wells released huge amounts of soot and toxic fumes into the atmosphere and might have had an impact on local weather patterns.

Global Warming

Many scientists predict that global warming could lead to a number of environmental problems, including drought, famine, wildfires, a rise in sea level, outbreaks of disease, and numerous environmental refugees.

Did you know?

- Of the hottest 20 years on record, 9 have occurred since 1980.
- The number of category 4 and 5 hurricanes worldwide has nearly doubled over the past 30 years.
- Fatal heat waves are becoming more frequent: at least 179 people died in the heat wave of 2006, and about 52,000 people died in the heat wave that struck Europe in 2003.
- One-third of all amphibian species are at risk of extinction due to global warming.
- Entire villages are being relocated in Alaska because the sea ice can no longer support them.

Global warming is the gradual increase in Earth's temperature. The **ozone layer**, part of Earth's stratosphere, protects the planet from the sun's UVB radiation. In the 1970s, researchers discovered that chlorofluorocarbons (CFCs) were contributing to the rapid depletion of the ozone layer. Earth's average surface temperature has risen by 1° F in the past century, with an accelerated increase over the past two decades.

Recently, scientists have discovered the first unequivocal link between the emission of human-made greenhouse gases and the dramatic heating of the oceans on Earth. They have explained a strong correlation between the rise in ocean temperatures over the past 40 years and the pollution of the atmosphere. These scientists have predicted that sea levels around the world could rise by more than 20 feet, with significant loss of shelf ice in Greenland and Antarctica, which would devastate coastal areas around the world. Other warnings include increased frequency and intensity of heat waves, and more frequent droughts and wildfires. Some scientists even believe that by 2050, the Arctic Ocean might have no ice during the summer by 2050, and that more than one million species worldwide could become extinct as a result of global warming.

Greenhouse gases include carbon dioxide, chlorofluorocarbons, ground-level ozone, nitrous oxide, and methane. These substances form a layer of gases that allow heat from the sun to pass through the atmosphere to Earth but traps the heat as it rises from Earth's surface.

CFC, or chlorofluorocarbons, is the collective name for compounds made of carbon, fluorine, chlorine, and hydrogen. Because they have stable, harmless, and noncombustible properties, these compounds are widely used in everyday products, such as coolants for air conditioners, cleaning agents for electronic components, and foaming agents for the manufacture of insulating materials.

Carbon dioxide and other gases naturally warm the surface of Earth by trapping heat from the sun in the atmosphere. The burning of fossil fuels, such as coal, natural gas, and oil, and the clearing of forests has dramatically increased the amount of carbon dioxide in Earth's atmosphere. As a result, global temperatures are rising, glaciers are melting, polar bears are drowning, plants and animals are being forced to leave their habitats, and the frequency of severe storms and droughts is increasing.

Global warming is largely caused by pollution, which is caused by generating and using energy, including electricity from power plants, gasoline in the tanks of cars and trucks, and industrial consumption of coal, oil, and natural gas. Government handouts to big energy companies are responsible for the burning of ever more coal, oil, and natural gas. The problem of global warming requires multiple solutions, including strong governmental regulations and the effective enforcement of such regulations.

As mentioned earlier, Earth's climate has warmed by about 1° F since 1900. Scientists have shown that at least 279 species of plants and animals have responded to this level of global warming by moving closer to the poles. Most regions of the Arctic have experienced a rise in temperature of 4 to 7° F in the past 50 years. These changes are threatening the lives of animals such as polar bears, which live and hunt on the sea ice. Over the past 15 years, polar bears have experienced about a 15 percent decline in the number of offspring and a similar decrease in weight. If the Arctic sea ice begins to melt completely during the summer by 2050, as some scientists predict, polar bears as a species will have little chance of surviving.

Corals are in danger as well. Not only are coral reefs a beautiful and essential part of the environment, but they also provide protection to coastal areas against storm surges and tsunamis. Some coral species are facing the greatest threat to their survival in 500,000 years. According to a report for the Pew Center on Global Climate Change, one-fourth of the world's coral reefs have already been destroyed. Another study, one by the IUCN-World Conservation Union, warns that half of the existing corals on Earth could be eliminated by the year 2045, when average temperatures are predicted to be as much as 3° F higher than they currently are.

Hurricane Sandy

In 2012 Hurricane Sandy destroyed parts of New York and New Jersey with a sum of over $65 billion in clean up across the U.S. Climate scientists say that climate change may well have played an important role in the destruction caused by Sandy not just due to global warming but also to rising sea levels and warmer ocean temperatures off the northeast. Sandy was also affected by rapid warming far to the north in the Arctic. Cold Arctic air coming from one of these large dips in the jet stream to the west strengthened the storm, while a huge high pressure system to the north blocked Sandy's movement over the Atlantic and drove it directly into the east coast.

A 2012 report by the U.N. Intergovernmental Panel on Climate Change (IPCC) found that sea level rise has likely increased extreme coastal high water events around the world. By warming the seas and the atmosphere, global warming is also expected to alter hurricane frequency and strength, making North Atlantic hurricanes slightly more powerful, while reducing the overall number of storms during the coming decades.

Air Pollution

Air pollution is the contamination of the air by substances in amounts great enough to affect human safety, health, and comfort. Major sources of outdoor air pollution include emissions given off by transportation vehicles, electric power plants fueled by oil and coal, and industries.

Acid rain is the depositing on Earth's surface of sulfuric and nitrous acids absorbed from the atmosphere during the formation of rain droplets. Acid rain can damage vegetation as well as the ecosystems of lakes, rivers, and streams.

The ozone layer, as described earlier, plays an important role in protecting life on Earth by absorbing harmful ultraviolet radiation (UVB) from the sun. The ozone layer's depletion is global. A large ozone hole has been observed in the Antarctic Circle. Destruction of the ozone allows a greater amount of harmful ultraviolet radiation (UVB) to reach Earth's surface, which can result in increased cases of skin cancer and visual health concerns, such as cataracts.

Photochemical_smog is a secondary air pollutant that is created when primary pollutants react with sunlight and atmospheric oxygen. Denver, Los Angeles, Phoenix, and Salt Lake City are among the cities in the United States that experience the highest levels of photochemical smog.

Air pollutants also exist indoors. These pollutants are gases or particles of matter inside buildings and are harmful to human health. Some examples of indoor air pollution include asbestos, biogenic pollutants, combustion by-products, formaldehyde, radon, tobacco smoke, and volatile organic compounds.

Environmental Change	Health Effects
Ozone depletion	Skin cancer, cataracts
Temperature extremes	Heat stroke, malaria, malnutrition
Decreased precipitation resulting in droughts	Malnutrition, asthma, allergies, respiratory diseases
Increased frequency of floods and hurricanes	Cholera, diarrheal diseases, malnutrition, death

Health Effects of Global Environmental Change

Other Environment Diseases:

1. **Lead** is a harmful toxin and the major environmental hazard for children. Lead is a naturally occurring element that is used in the manufacture of many industrial and household products. Power plants and other industrial facilities emit lead into the air, where it eventually settles into the soil and dust. This lead is then brought into homes or ingested by children as they play outdoors and put their hands in their mouths. Very young children are particularly at risk of lead poisoning by putting pieces of lead paint peeling from walls into their mouths. Recent investigations have revealed that many toys, especially those made in China, are contaminated with lead. Health problems associated with lead include anemia, birth defects, and bone and neurological damage. For children, even small amounts of lead have been shown to lower IQ levels.

   Solutions for the prevention of lead poisoning include education, regulation of the use of lead, and individual responsibility for knowing what materials contain lead and avoiding using or coming in contact with them.

   Prevention of Lead Poisoning includes the following:
   - **Avoid direct contact with soil,** especially if you live in an urban area or near a highway.
   - **Wash your hands as soon as you get home from work.**
   - **Take your shoes off at the door** to avoid bringing contaminated soil into the home.
   - **Vacuum carpets frequently** using an HEPA vacuum cleaner. Use a damp rag frequently to clean painted wooden windowsills, moldings, and floors.
   - **Check for peeling or flaking paint,** especially if your home was built before 1978. Have the paint tested by a professional service or with a home testing kit.
   - **Test imported dishware or pottery** before cooking or serving food in it. Lead paints and glazes are still used outside the United States and Europe. Lead-contaminated dishes and pottery—particularly from Mexico and China—have recently been found in stores in the United States.
   - **Avoid toys imported from China.**
   - **Let tap water run for a few minutes** before you drink it to make sure that any water that has been standing in the pipes has run through.
   - **Use charcoal filters for water, including filters for pitchers.**

2. **Malaria** is a disease caused by mosquitoes and transmitted from person to person. It kills between one and two million people annually, mainly in tropical parts of Africa, and debilitates as many as 400 million others. Scientists believe that climate is the major factor in the spread of malaria, because mosquitoes live in warm, humid environments. In warm regions of the world other than Africa, methods of repelling and killing mosquitoes, including netting and mass-spraying of pesticides, are largely responsible for limiting the incidences of malaria.

3. **Asthma** is a chronic, inflammatory lung disease with symptoms that include recurring episodes of breathlessness, wheezing, coughing, and chest tightness. These episodes are known as exacerbations or attacks. National data indicate that the number of children who have asthma in the United States has more than doubled in the past 15 years. Asthma is a growing concern especially for African-American and Latino children who live in inner-cities. Estimates indicate that one out of four African American children living in New York City has asthma. African-American children age 4 and younger are six times as likely as white children of similar ages to die from asthma, and even those who escape death are hospitalized more often than are white children. In other developed countries, the number of children who are diagnosed with asthma has also increased significantly. Most scientists attribute this rise in the incidence of childhood asthma on air pollution. The environment is a major factor in the onset and severity of asthma.

Chemicals and biological agents that increase the risk of an asthma attack include the following:

- Second-hand smoke from cigarettes, especially in indoor environments, brings on asthma attacks in many people who are sensitive, and it may be a cause in the development of asthma in younger children.

- Allergens produced by dust mites, cockroaches, mold, and pets in homes can trigger wheezing and other symptoms of asthma in those who are allergic to them.

- Exposure to ozone or diesel exhaust exacerbates the effects of allergies on asthma, but about 99 percent of U.S. school buses run on diesel fuel.

Other factors that contribute to the development and exacerbation of asthma include living in poor housing conditions, living in urban areas near high-traffic roads, and lack of access to adequate medical care.

What do hamburgers have to do with the environment?

It is widely known that industrial farms illegally dump millions of tons of untreated fecal and toxic waste onto land and into water. This type of farming has contaminated numerous bodies of water, killed billions of fish and other organisms, sickened consumers, and subjected millions of animals to cruel treatment.

Cattle emit huge volumes of methane, a gas that is 23 times more efficient in trapping heat than carbon dioxide. The manure of cattle bred for meat is the source of two-thirds of human-caused nitrous oxide, a greenhouse gas that is 300 times as potent as carbon dioxide. The farming of corn, soybeans, and hay for livestock feed accounts for about half of all fertilizers used in the United States, and generates large amounts of nitrous oxide. In Brazil, thousands of acres of rain forests are being cut down to clear the land for pastures and fields in which to grow animal feed.

One solution that individuals can participate in to reduce global environmental changes is to eat less meat and more whole foods, such as beans, nuts, fruits, and vegetables. Such a diet also reduces the risk of obesity, diabetes, and heart disease.

Water

Water is a necessity for all forms of life, yet access to safe and clean drinking water is a huge concern for many people around the world. Only about 3 percent of the water on Earth is freshwater, and two-thirds of that water is unavailable in glaciers. The main sources of freshwater are rainwater; surface water from streams, lakes, and rivers; and groundwater.

A person can survive for a month or longer without food but only for about three days without water. Thousands of chemicals that are used in industrial processes, as well as lead, sewage, and gasoline have been found in tap water in the United States. It is safest to drink charcoal-filtered water, water that has been boiled (which still does not eliminate lead), or bottled spring water.

All tap water has chemicals added to it, specifically chlorine and fluoride. Some scientists believe that these chemicals cause high levels of toxicity, which can scar the arteries. Fluoride affects the thyroid gland. The United States has the highest levels of fluoride in tap water and and the highest obesity rate in the world. Fluoride has been linked to depression and physical problems, some related to thyroid activity and possibly even obesity. Chlorine is a poison, and high doses of it kills living organisms.

The U.S. Environmental Protection Agency (EPA) routinely assures the public that nearly 100 percent of community water systems meet clean drinking water standards. However, in a test by the Environmental Working Group of tap water from a variety of cities, the group found 119 "normal" chemicals (those for which the EPA allows in water but has set limits) and another 141 chemicals that are completely unregulated.

Water quality in the U.S. is threatened by four conditions:

1. Population growth
2. Growth of the chemical industry
3. Environmental mismanagement, including irresponsible disposal of wastes
4. Reckless land-use practices

Chemical water pollution typically occurs for the following reasons:

- Chemicals dumped into the water intentionally
- Chemicals seep into groundwater, streams, or rivers through leaky pipes or storage tanks
- Chemicals contaminate bodies of water as a result of industrial accidents
- Pollution is cycled from polluted air through rainwater
- Chemicals can leach out of contaminated soil

The types of chemical contamination described above are called **point sources** of water pollution. **Non-point-sources** are sources that cause pollution of water secondhand, such as pesticide runoff from farm fields and lawns, as well as runoff of automotive fluids and other chemicals from roads, parking lots, driveways, and other surfaces, which flow into bodies of water or seep into groundwater.

Biological hazards include organisms that are harmful to humans, such as water-borne diseases that are transmitted through drinking water. Examples of biological hazards include the polio virus, the hepatitis A virus, salmonella, shigella, cholera, amoebic dysentery, and cryptosporidium. These disease-causing organisms are transported into water from feces, and can cause illnesses in people who drink or cook with this untreated, contaminated water.

Pesticides are chemicals that are manufactured to destroy pests. Pesticides include herbicides and insecticides. The misuse or overuse of pesticides can result in illness and even death in humans.

The best-known case of pesticide pollution in the United States occurred in the 1960s, when the insecticide DDT was found to have polluted waterways, which then contaminated fish and poisoned animals that ate the fish. DDT was banned from agricultural use in the U.S. in 1972 and shortly thereafter was banned worldwide at the Stockholm Convention after concerns were raised, largely as a result of the research and efforts of biologist Rachael Carson, over its effects on the environment, and on animal and human health. DDT was alleged to be a liver and breast carcinogen, and women who were exposed to the pesticide were found to have higher than normal rates of infertility. However, DDT it is still used in some developing countries to destroy malaria-carrying mosquitoes. Many Americans continue to be exposed to DDT through produce that was grown in tropical countries, as well as through fish caught in some U.S. waters.

In terms of general human health, pesticides can have the following effects:

- Damage the nervous system
- Liver damage
- Damage DNA and cause a variety of cancers
- Reproductive and endocrine damage

Water Bottles

Bottled water produces up to 1.5 million tons of plastic waste per year. Rather than being recycled, about 75 percent of the empty plastic bottles end up in our landfills, lakes, streams, and oceans, where they may never fully decompose. According to Food and Water Watch, that type of plastic requires up to 47 million gallons of oil per year to produce. And while the plastic used to bottle beverages is of high quality and in demand by recyclers, over 80 percent of plastic bottles are simply thrown away. Plastic waste now ends up in the world's major oceans, which is devastating to marine life, killing birds and fish.

Intersex Fish

Many of the chemicals that are dumped into waterways in the United States disrupt hormones. These chemicals cause interrupted sexual development in fish in water with high hormone concentrations; that is, female fish begin to exhibit male fish characteristics and vice versa.

Other effects on fish include thyroid system disorders, the inability to breed, weakened immune responses, and abnormal mating and other behaviors. In humans, hormone disruptors lead to weakened immune functions, mental impairments, increases in the incidences of infertility, and increases in the development of some types of cancers.

Chemicals that can make you FAT:

Obesogens are chemicals that can disrupt your hormonal balance and can make you fat. They are also referred to as endocrine disruptors.

Here are the Top 5:

1. Bisphenol-A (BPA) – Found in baby bottles, plastics, and canned foods and associated with obesity and cancer.
2. Phthalates – Chemicals found in many plastics, associated with abdominal obesity and genital malformations in boys.
3. Atrazine – A herbicide in common use in the U.S., associated with birth defects, mitochondrial damage, and obesity.
4. Organotins – Chemicals used as fungicides, linked to weight gain and fatty liver disease in mice.
5. Perfluorooctanoic Acid (PFOA) – A compound found in non-stick cookware, associated with cancer and fat gain.

To avoid these chemicals:

1. Eat organic food.
2. Avoid foods and beverages that have been stored in plastic containers.
3. Use stainless steel or quality aluminum water bottles instead of plastic.
4. Do NOT feed your babies from plastic bottles. Use glass bottles instead.
5. Instead of non-stick cookware, use cast iron, ceramic, or stainless steel.
6. Use organic, natural cosmetics.

What Can You Do to Help the Environment?

With less than 5 percent of the world's population, the United States produces between one-fifth and one-fourth of the world's greenhouse-gas emissions.

In addition, more than 100 million trees are cut down every year to produce junk mail, not to mention the 28 billion gallons of water that are used for this purpose. The energy resources annually used to produce and dispose of junk mail exceeds the amount used to power 2.8 million cars.

Conserve Energy

People can conserve energy by driving hybrid cars, using public transportation, installing solar panels in their homes, and using fluorescent light bulbs. People can also lobby companies to stop sending unsolicited junk mail and catalogs, which contribute to the destruction of the rain forests.

Reduce Pollution

Individuals and groups can help to develop national strategies and policies to address air pollution. They also can support policies that encourage the use of renewable resources, and use and support alternative methods of transportation. Most experts agree that alternative methods of transportation are necessary to reduce air pollution significantly.

Stop the Destruction of Rain Forests

The most recent estimates indicate that approximately 150,000 square kilometers of tropical rain forests, roughly equal to the size of England and Wales combined, is destroyed every year. Rain forests are valuable for a variety of reasons. First, they continuously recycle carbon dioxide into oxygen. In fact, more than 20 percent of the world's oxygen is produced in the Amazon Rain Forest, followed by the Congo of Central Africa, which is the second-largest rain forest on Earth. Millions of people depend on the rain forests for their survival, and obtain food, medicine, and shelter there. The rain forests are also essential in the regulation of local and global climates. Thus, it is important that people make every effort to stop the destruction of the rain forests.

Rain forests are destroyed because they are:

- Rich in minerals, including oil, gold, aluminum, iron, and cobalt
- Used for seismic testing for oil
- Used by the logging industry
- Used for the cutting of tracks and routes for oil pipelines
- Used for commercial and subsistence farming
- Used by huge plantations of rubber trees, within which bananas, soy beans, and oil palms are also grown
- Used for the production of paper

Scientists estimate that nearly half of the world's species of plants, animals, and microorganisms will be destroyed or threatened over several decades as a result of rain forest destruction. As their homelands continue to be destroyed by deforestation, indigenous rain forest peoples are also disappearing. Five hundred years ago, an estimated 10 million Native Peoples lived in the Amazonian Rain Forest, while today, there are less than 200,000. If deforestation continues at current rates, scientists estimate that between 80 and 90 percent of the tropical rain forests' ecosystems could be destroyed by the year 2020.

Simple Ways You Can Improve Earth's Health

Environmental scientists warn that global warming will affect every person, community, and nation, creating a cycle of events likely to have harmful results. People's choices about where to live, work, travel, and what to buy have a profound effect on their health and on the health of others around the world. The following are ways in which individuals can make a positive impact on the environment:

- Switch to highly efficient compact fluorescent light bulbs (CFLs) that last for years, use only one-fourth of the energy of regular light bulbs, and actually produce more light.

- Buy a fuel-efficient car, such as a hybrid. Replacing gas-guzzling cars with fuel-efficient ones is by far the most important contribution that an individual can make. Although automakers haven't yet sold enough hybrids in the United States to make them as affordable as they should be, this will change if there is a demand for more hybrids and less for the gas guzzlers.
- Turn off equipment such as televisions and stereos when they are not in use. The little red standby light means that they are still using power and that means a contribution to global warming.
- Conserve water by turning off the tap while brushing your teeth and by collecting the water used to wash vegetables and salad greens to water houseplants.
- Call 311 to find a disposal location for used car batteries, cell phones, and other hazardous household waste items.
- Recycle paper, glass, plastics, and other waste.
- Use rechargeable batteries.
- Don't use "throw-away" products such as paper plates and napkins, or plastic knives, forks, and cups, because these contribute to more garbage.
- Celebrate Earth Day by organizing and participating in protests to preserve our land.
- Work to find alternative energy sources.
- Elect officials who fight against corporate polluters, not give them tax breaks.

References:

Amoco Cadiz, http://greennature.com/article219.html.

Arctic Climate Impact Assessment. *Impacts of a Warming Arctic*, Cambridge: Cambridge University Press, 2004. Also quoted in *Time Magazine*, "Vicious Cycles," Missy Adams, March 26, 2006.

Bjerklie, David. "Feeling the Heat," *Time Magazine*, March 26, 2006.

Carson, Rachel. *Silent Spring*, Portland, OR: Mariner Books, 2002.

Chernobyl, at http://www.chernobyl.co.uk/ and the Chernobyl Children's Project International, at http://www.chernobyl-international.com/aboutchernobyl/disaster.asp.

Colborn, T. "Pesticides—How research has succeeded and failed to translate science into policy: Endocrinological effects on wildlife," *Environmental Health Perspectives Supplements* 103 (Suppl 6) (1995): 81-86.

Conin, John and Kennedy, Robert Jr. *The Riverkeeper: Two Activists Fight to Reclaim Our Environment as a Basic Human Right*, 1st Touchstone ed., BC, Canada: Scribner, 1999.

Columbia University. World Trade Center Environmental Contaminant Database (WTCECD) New York: Mailman School of Public Health, Columbia University, 2003. Available at http://wtc.hs.columbia.edu/wtc/.

Dejmek J., Selevan, S.G., Benes, I., Solansky, I., and Sram, R.J. "Fetal growth and maternal exposure to particulate matter during pregnancy," *Environ Health Perspect* 107 (1999): 475-480.

Diamond, J. *Collapse: How Societies Choose to Fail or Succeed*, New York: Viking, 2005.

Dodson, R.F., Williams, M.G., Corn, C.J., Brollo, A., and Bianchi, C. "A comparison of asbestos burden in lung parenchma, lymph nodes and plaques," *Ann NY Acad Sci* 643 (1991): 53-60.

Edelman P., Osterloh, J., Pirkle, J., Caudill, S.P., Grainger, J., Jones, R., et al. "Biomonitoring of chemical exposure among New York City firefighters responding to the World Trade Center fire and collapse," *Environ Health Perspect* 111 (2003): 1906-1911.

Eilperin, J. "Debate on Climate Shifts to Issue of Irreparable Change," *The Washington Post*, January 29, 2006, A1.

Emanuel, K. "Increasing destructiveness of tropical cyclones over the past 30 years," *Nature* 436 (2005): 686-688.

ENDS. "Pesticides in drinking water linked to breast cancer," ENDS Report 241 (1995): 8-9.

Fairbrother, G., Stuber, J., Galea, S., Fleischman, A.R., and Pfefferbaum, B. "Post-traumatic stress reactions in New York City children after the September 11, 2001, terrorist attacks," *Ambul Pediatrics* 3 (2003): 304-311.

Galea, S., Ahern, J., Resnick, H., Kilpatrick, D., Bucuvalas, M., Gold, J., et al. "Psychological sequelae of the September 11 terrorist attacks in New York City," *N Engl J Med* 346 (2002): 982-987.

Galea, S., Resnick, H., Ahern, J., Gold, J., Bucuvalas, M., Kilpatrick, D., et al. (2002b). "Post-traumatic stress disorder in Manhattan, New York City, after the September 11th terrorist attacks," *J Urban Health* 79 (2002): 340-353.

Gavett, S.H., Haykal-Coates, N., Highfill, J.W., Ledbetter, A.D., Chen, L.C., Cohen, M.D., et al. "World Trade Center fine particulate matter causes respiratory tract hyperresponsiveness in mice," *Environ Health Perspect* 111 (2003): 981-991.

Gibbs, Lois Marie. *Love Canal: The Story Continues*, 20 anniv. ed. BC, Canada: New Society Publishers, 1998.

Gore, Al. *An Inconvenient Truth: The Planetary Emergency of Global Warming and What We Can Do About It*, New York, NY: Rodale Books, 2006.

http:// www.nasa.gov.

http:// www.pewclimate.org.

http://www.washingtonpost.com/2006/08/03.

http://news.nationalgeographic.com/2006.

http://www.arctic.noaa.gov.

Institute for Environment and Health. "Environmental oestrogens: Consequences to human health and wildlife," Leicester: University of Leicester, 1995.

Jacobson, S.W., Jacobson, J.L., O'Neill, J.M., Padgett, R.J., Frankowski, J.J., and Bihun, J.T. "Visual expectation and dimensions of infant information processing," *Child Dev* 63 (1992): 711-724.

Kennedy, Robert Jr. *Crimes Against Nature: How George W. Bush and His Corporate Pals Are Plundering the Country and Hijacking Our Democracy*, New York, NY: Harper Perennial, 2005.

Kennedy, Robert Jr. "Crimes Against Nature," *Rolling Stone Magazine*, December 11, 2003.

Kogevinas, M. "Human health effects of dioxins: cancer, reproductive and endocrine system effects," *Hum Reprod* 7 (2001): 331-339.

Krabill, W., Hanna, E., Huybrechts, P., Abdalati, W., Cappelen, J., Csatho, B., Frefick, E., Manizade, S., Martin, C., Sonntag, J., Swift, R., Thomas, R., and Yungel, J. "Greenland Ice Sheet: Increased coastal thinning," *Geophysical Research Letters* 31 (2004).

Kelce, W.R., Stone, C.R., Laws, S.C., Gray, L.E., Kemppainen, J.A., and Wilson, E.M. "Persistent DDT metabolite p, p'-DDE is a potent androgen receptor antagonist," *Nature* 375 (1995): 581-585.

Landrigan, P.J. "Health consequences of the 11 September 2001 attacks," *Environ Health Perspect* 109 (2001): A514-A515.

LeBouffant, L., Martin, J.C., Durif, W., and Daniel, H. "Structure and composition of pleural plaque," *IARC Sci Publ* 8 (1973): 249-257.

LeBlanc, G.A. "Are environmental sentinels signaling?" *Environ. Health Perspective* 103 (1995): 888-890.

Levin S., Herbert, R., Skloot, G., Szeinuk, J., Teirstein, A., Fischler, D., et al. "Health effects of World Trade Center site workers," *Am J Ind Med* 42 (2001): 545-547.

Lioy, P.J., Weisel, C.P., Millette, J.R., Eisenreich, S., Vallero, D., Offenberg, J., et al. Characterization of the dust/smoke aerosol that settled east of the World Trade Center (WTC) in Lower Manhattan after the collapse of the WTC 11 September 2001," *Environ Health Perspect* 110 (2002): 703-714.

Lippy, B.E. "Safety and health of heavy equipment operators at Ground Zero," *Am J Ind Med* 42 (2002): 539-542.

Lomborg, B. *The Skeptical Environmentalist—Measuring the Real State of the World*, Cambridge: Cambridge University Press, 1998.

Maynard, R. "Sperm alert," *Living Earth* 188 (995): 8-9.

McKinney, M.L. and Schoch, R.M. *Environmental Science: Systems and Solutions*, 3rd ed. Sudbury, Massachusetts: Jones and Bartlett, 2003.

Magnani, C., Dalmasso, P., Biggeri, A., Ivaldi, C., Mirabelli, D., and Terracini, B. "Increased risk of malignant mesothelioma of the pleura after residential or domestic exposure to asbestos: a case-control study in Casale Monferrato, Ital," *Environ Health Perspect* 109 (2001): 915-919.

Malievskaya, E., Rosenberg, N., and Markowitz, S. "Assessing the health of immigrant workers near Ground Zero: preliminary results of the World Trade Center Day Laborer Medical Monitoring Project," *Am J Ind Med* 42 (2002): 548-549.

McCurdy, T., Glen, G., Smith, L., and Lakkadi, Y. "The national exposure research laboratory's consolidated human activity database," *J Expo Anal Environ Epidemiol* 10(6 Pt 1) (2000): 566-578.

McGee, J.K., Chen, L.C., Cohen, M.D., Chee, G.R., Prophete, C.M., Haykal-Coates, N., et al. "Chemical analysis of World Trade Center fine particulate matter for use in toxicological assessment," *Environ Health Perspect* 111 (2003): 972-980.

Nicholson, W.J. and Landrigan, P.J. "Asbestos: A status report," *Curr Issues Public Health* 2 (1996): 118-123.

Nicholson, W.J., Rohl, A.N., Ferrand, E.F. "Asbestos air pollution in New York City," in *Proceedings of the Second International Clean Air Congress*, Englund, H.M, & Beery, W.T., eds. New York: Academic Press, 1971, 36-139.

NOAA Oil Spill Review, 2003, at http://response.restoration.noaa.gov/oilaids/spilldb.pdf.

Offenberg, J.H., Eisenreich, S.J., Chen, L.C., Cohen, M.D., Chee, G., Prophete, C., et al. "Persistent organic pollutants in the dusts that settled across lower Manhattan after September 11, 2001," *Environ Sci Technol* 37 (2003): 502-508.

Perera, F.P., Whyatt, R.M., Jedrychowski, W., Rauh, V., Manchester, D., Santella, R.M., et al. "Recent developments in molecular epidemiology: A study of the effects of environmental polycyclic aromatic hydrocarbons on birth outcomes in Poland," *Am J Epidemiol* 147 (1998): 309-314.

Prezant, D.J., Weiden, M., Banauch, G.I., McGuinness, G., Rom, W.N., and Aldrich, T.K. "Cough and bronchial responsiveness in firefighters at the World Trade Center site," *N Engl J Med* 347 (2002): 806-815.

Pruss-Ustun A. and Corvalen C. "Preventing disease through healthy environments: Toward an estimate of the environmental burden of disease," Geneva: World Health Organization, 2006.

Reibman, J., Lin, S., Matte, T., Rogers, L., Hoerning, A., Hwang, S., et al. "Respiratory health of residents near the former World Trade Center: The WTC Residents Respiratory Health Survey" (abstract), *Am J Respir Crit Care Med* 167 (2003): A335.

Reitze, W.B., Nicholson, W.J., Holaday, D.A., and Selikoff, I.J. "Application of sprayed inorganic fiber containing asbestos: Occupational health hazards," *Am Ind Hyg Assoc J* 33 (1972): 178-191.

Ritz, B., Yu, F., Chapa, G., and Fruin, S. "Effect of air pollution on preterm birth among children born in Southern California between 1989 and 1993," *Epidemiology* 11 (2000): 502-511.

Rom, W.N., Weiden, M., Garcia, R., Yie, T.A., Vathesatogkit, P., Tse, D.B., et al. "Acute eosinophilic pneumonia in a New York City firefighter exposed to World Trade Center dust," *Am J Respir Crit Care Med* 166 (2002): 797-800.

Scanlon, M.D. "World Trade Center cough—A lingering legacy and a cautionary tale," *N Engl J Med* 347 (2002): 840-842.

Schlenger, W.E., Caddell, J.M., Ebert, L., Jordan, B.K., Rourke, K.M., Wilson, D., et al. "Psychological reactions to terrorist attacks: Findings from the National Study of Americans' Reactions to September 11," *JAMA* 288 (2002): 581-588.

Sharpe, R. M. "Another DDT connection," *Nature* 375 (1995): 538-539.

Shepherd, P.A. and Fagan, J.F. *The Fagan Test of Infant Intelligence*, Cleveland: Infantest Corp., 1987.

Soto, A.M., Sonnenschein, C., Chung, K.L., Fernandez, M.F., Olea, N., and Serrano, F.O. "The E-SCREEN assay as a tool to identify estrogens: An update on estrogenic environmental pollutants," *Environ. Health Perspect* 103 (suppl. 7) (1995): 113-122.

Spadafora, R. "Firefighter safety and health issues at the Word Trade Center site," *Am J Ind Med* 42 (2002): 532-538.

Stuber, J., Fairbrother, G., Galea, S., Pfefferbaum, B., Wilson-Genderson, M., and Vlahov, D. "Determinants of counseling for children in Manhattan after the September 11 attacks," *Psychiatr Serv* 53 (2002): 815-822.

Suzuki, Y. and Yuen, S.R. "Asbestos fibers contributing to the induction of human malignant mesothelioma," Annals, *NY Acad Sci* 982 (2002): 160-176.

Taylor, Leslie. *The Healing Power of Rainforest Herbs*, New York: Square One Publishers, 2004.

Thurston, G. and Chen, L.C. "Risk communication in the aftermath of the World Trade Center disaster," *Am J Ind Med* 42 (2002): 543-544.

Thurston, G., Maciejczyk, P., Lall, R., Hwang, J., and Chen, L.C. "Identification and characterization of World Trade Center Disaster fine particulate matter air pollution at a site in Lower Manhattan following September 11," *Epidemiology* 14 (2003): S87-S88.

U.S. Department of Labor. *Asbestos*, 2003, at http://www.osha.gov/SLTC/asbestos/.

U.S. Environmental Protection Agency. *Asbestos Hazard Emergency Response Act (AHERA): Region 2 Compliance*, 1986, at http://www.epa.gov/region02/ahera/ahera.htm.

U.S. Environmental Protection Agency. *Exposure and Human Health Evaluation of Airborne Pollution from the World Trade Center Disaster* (External Review Draft), EPA/600/P-2/002A, Washington, D.C.: Environmental Protection Agency, 2002.

U.S. Environmental Protection Agency, at http://www.epa.gov/ncea/wtc.htm.

U.S. Environmental Protection Agency. "Toxicological Effects of Fine Particulate Matter Derived from the Destruction of the World Trade Center," *Fact Sheet: Release of Reports Related to the World Trade Center Disaster: Exposure and Human Health Evaluation of Airborne Pollution from the World Trade Center Disaster*, Washington, D.C.: Environmental Protection Agency, 2003.

U.S. Environmental Protection Agency. *EPA Response to September 11*, Washington, D.C.: Environmental Protection Agency, 2004, at http://www.epa.gov/wtc/.

Vlahov, D., Galea, S., and Frankel, D. "New York City, 2001: Reaction and response," *J Urban Health* 79 (2002): 2-5.

Vlahov, D., Galea, S., Resnick, H., Ahern, J., Boscarino, J.A., Bucuvalas, M, et al. "Increased use of cigarettes, alcohol, and marijuana among Manhattan, New York, residents after the September 11th terrorist attacks," *Am J Epidemiol* 155 (2002): 988-996.

World Health Organization, at www.who.gov/environmentalhealth.

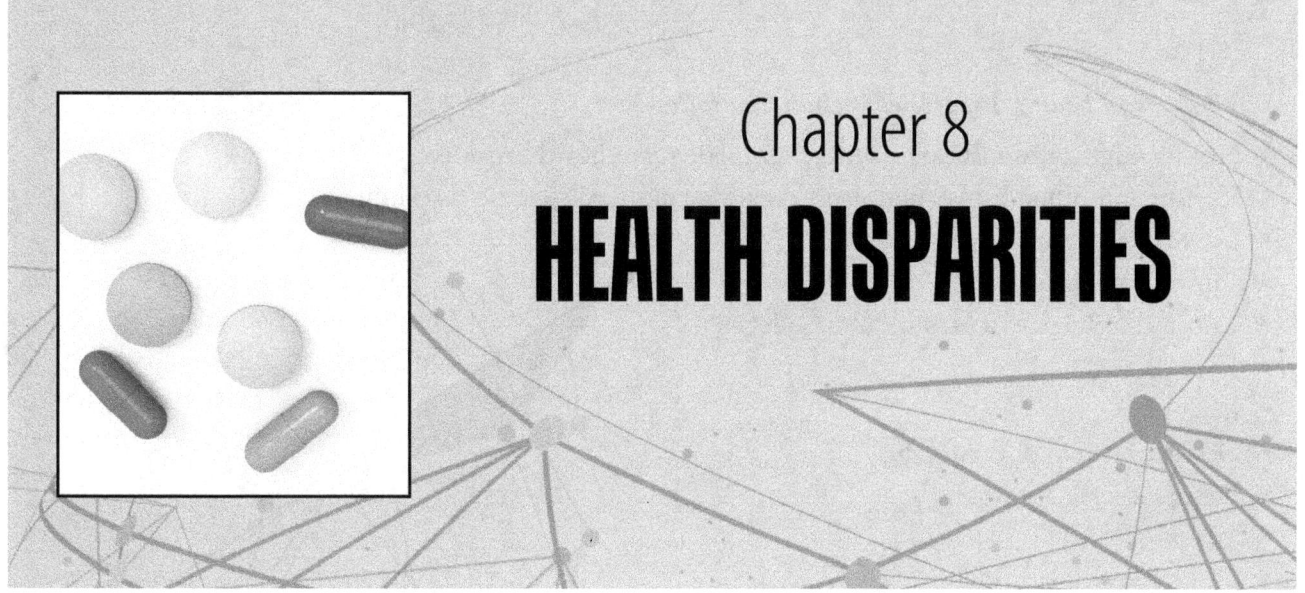

Chapter 8
HEALTH DISPARITIES

The greatest single challenge facing our globalized
world is to combat and eradicate its disparities.

—*Nelson Mandela*

Cultural, ethnic, and racial diversity remains one of the strengths of the United States as our population continues to grow. However, there are significant disparities in health between various minorities and the general population. Inequalities in health are based upon observable differences, or disparities, in the health of different populations.

Health disparities are differences in the occurrences, prevalence, mortality, and burden of diseases, as well as other detrimental health conditions that exist among specific population groups. Such disparities occur when a group, whether it is defined by a gender, race, ethnicity, or community, has a higher predisposition for disease or illness than does the larger population to which it belongs.

When there is a significant difference in the overall rate of incidences and prevalence of disease, morbidity, mortality, or survival rates in a specific part of a population in comparison with the health status of the general population, a **health disparity population** exists.

An example of a health disparity is the **infant mortality rate**, which is the number of children who die before they reach age 1 divided by the number of live births that year. The infant mortality rate is the most significant measure of the well being of infants in any given population.

Factors that influence an infant mortality rate include the following:

- The health of the mother
- Quality of and access to medical care
- Socioeconomic conditions
- Environmental conditions
- Public health practices

In the United States, the infant mortality rate of whites is 5.9 per 1,000, whereas the rate for African-Americans is 13.9 per 1,000. The difference between the two rates clearly indicates that there are health disparities between these two groups in the overall population.

Contributors to health disparities include the following:

- Not having health insurance or having inadequate health insurance
- Racism and other "isms" that decrease opportunities or cause discrimination
- Lack of transportation
- Lifestyle behaviors
- Cultural influences, customs, and beliefs
- Poor diet
- Lack of exercise
- Obesity or being overweight
- Unsafe sexual behavior
- Stress
- Mental health issues
- Systemic barriers
- Access to health care
- Poverty
- Environmental factors

Diversity Mantra: (Oxford University)
➤ Just because *you* see it that way, doesn't mean everyone does.
➤ Just because *you* learn best that way, doesn't mean everyone does.
➤ Just because *you* like it that way, doesn't mean everyone does.

Why is Diversity Significant?

By the year 2050, nearly half of the U.S. population will be composed of racial minorities. As we move into the future, health care systems are and will continue to deal with a much more diverse and less healthy population. Health disparities in the United States are not new phenomena; they have existed throughout our history. Health disparities for ethnic and racial minorities continue to be a community problem, with not nearly enough progress having been made to eliminate them.

The most common health disparities known to exist in the United States relate to heart disease, cancer, diabetes, accidental injuries, and HIV/AIDS. According to former Surgeon General David Satcher, the mortality rate for heart disease is more than 40 percent higher for African Americans than for whites. The mortality rate for all types of cancer is 30 percent higher for African Americans than it is for whites, with African American women experiencing higher mortality rates from breast cancer, despite an increase in screening for this group. The incidence of prostate cancer for African American men is more than double that of white men. For African Americans, the rate of HIV/AIDS is more than seven times the rate for whites and, specifically for African American women, the incidence of HIV is as much as 20 times higher than it is for white women. As for homicide, the rate is six times higher for African Americans than it is for whites (cdc.gov/hiv/pubs/facts/women).

Causes of death that are highest among minorities in the U.S. include the following:

- **Infant mortality:** the highest predictor of overall health in a population (this is often a result of a lack of access to good prenatal care)
- **Cancer:** the rate of deaths is high due to a lack of screening
- **Cardiovascular disease and stroke:** both are caused by hypertension, obesity, poor diet, and unhealthful lifestyle behaviors
- **Diabetes type 2:** the result of a poor diet, obesity, and a sedentary lifestyle
- **Homicide and accidents:** these often result from poverty and negative social and/or living conditions
- **Chemical dependence:** often a result of low level of education and low income

Health disparities in the United States are most common among the four main ethnic or racial groups in this country: African Americans, Hispanics, Asian/Pacific Islanders, and Native Americans. Historically, these groups, as well as immigrants, the poor, and the mentally challenged, have not received the level of health care that the general population has, which is reflected by their high morbidity and mortality rates.

As we approach the year 2050, our nation will be increasingly more diverse, racial and ethnic minorities accounted for 91.7 percent of the nation's total growth between 2000 and 2010; non-Hispanic whites accounted for the remaining 8.3 percent.

African Americans

The U.S. Census Bureau projects that by the year 2060 there will be 77.4 million African Americans in the United States, making up 18.4 percent of the total U.S. population. However, this group experiences a disproportionate amount of diseases, injuries, death, and disabilities resulting from a variety of medical conditions as compared with other racial or ethnic groups and with the general population. Disparities in the socioeconomic status of African Americans as compared with whites include higher unemployment and underemployment, lower levels of education, discrimination, and more poverty among African Americans. All of these factors contribute significantly to disparities in their health status.

Health disparities between African Americans and whites include the following:

- African Americans have higher rates of morbidity and mortality for many chronic diseases that are associated with a poor diet and obesity.
- The mortality rate for cancer of African-American men is 1.4 times higher than it is for white men, and for African-American women, that rate is 1.2 times higher than it is for white women.
- The life expectancy of African Americans is lower than it is for whites.
- In 2009, high school completion among African American adults was the second lowest (second to completion among Hispanic adults and similar to the completion among American Indian/Alaska Native adults).
- In 2009, the percentage of African American adults living in poverty was among the largest compared with other racial/ethnic populations (similar to percentages among American Indians/Alaska Natives and Hispanic Americans).
- In 2009, African American adults more often lived in inadequate and unhealthy housing than White adults. The percentage of African American adults living in inadequate housing was similar to percentages among American Indian/Alaska Native and Hispanic adults. These populations had the largest percentages of adults living in inadequate housing.

- Sickle-cell anemia is another disease that disproportionately afflicts African Americans. An estimated 1 out of 12 African Americans is born with the sickle cell trait, and about 1 out of 375 is born with sickle cell anemia.

Sickle Cell Anemia

Sickle cell anemia is a disease in which the body manufactures sickle-shaped (or crescent-shaped) red blood cells instead of the normally C-shaped red blood cells. An abnormal hemoglobin level causes these cells to have their sickle shape, which prevents them from moving easily through the blood vessels. Instead of being smooth and able to glide easily, sickle cells are stiff and sticky, and they are prone to clumping and getting stuck in the blood vessels. When this happens, the clumps of sickle cells block the flow of blood that lead to the limbs and internal organs. Blood vessels that are blocked can cause pain, severe infections, and organ damage. Sickle cell anemia is an inherited, lifelong disease. People who have the disease are born with it. They inherit two copies of the sickle cell gene—one from each parent (NHLBI.gov).

Hispanics

Health disparities between Hispanics and non-Hispanic whites include the following:

- Mortality rates for accidents, homicide, and HIV/AIDS are higher for Americans of Hispanic origin than they are for non-Hispanic whites.
- Not only do Hispanics have higher mortality rates for diabetes than do non-Hispanic whites, but they are also twice as likely to die from this disease.
- Hispanics have higher rates of hypertension and obesity than do non-Hispanic whites.
  - Hispanic children have the highest childhood obesity rate in the country, with about two in five Hispanic children aged 2 to 19 being overweight or obese.
  - Latinas are twice as likely to die from pregnancy-associated complications as their white counterparts.
  - Latinos are also disproportionately affected by HIV/AIDS and are three times more likely than their white counterparts to be infected.
  - Latinas are 20% more likely to die from breast cancer than white women.
  - Latinos exceeded all other racial or ethnic groups with the largest percentage (29%) of reported tuberculosis cases in the United States in 2010.
- Half of all Latino children born in 2000 are at risk of developing diabetes

(Source: www.americanprogress.org)

For socioeconomic reasons, Hispanics as a group lag behind the general population in their levels of education. Both low levels of education and poverty contribute to the poorer health status of Hispanics as a group. In some cases, the immigration status of Hispanics leaves them with no access to health insurance and little access to health care.

Acculturation is the process by which immigrants adopt the attitudes, values, customs, beliefs, and behaviors of the culture in their new country. The **Hispanic Paradox** is a theory that states that immigrants of Hispanic origin are healthier before they come to the United States and then go on to acculturate and take up unhealthful habits that are common in this country.

Greater acculturation is associated with the following:

- Increased rate of infant mortality and low birth weight
- Overall cancer rates
- High blood pressure
- Adolescent pregnancies
- Smoking, alcohol consumption, and illicit drug use
- Decreased consumption of fiber
- Depression

Asian/Pacific Islanders

In 2011, the population of Asians, including those of more than one race, was estimated at 18.2 million in the U.S. population. The three largest Asian groups in the United States in 2011 were Chinese (4 million, except Taiwanese descent), Filipinos (3.4 million), and Asian Indians (3.2 million). These were followed by Vietnamese (1.9 million), Koreans (1.7 million), and Japanese (1.3 million). The U.S. Census Bureau projec that by the year 2050, there will be more than 40.6 million Asians living in the United States, comp ng 9.2 percent of the total U.S. population.

While Asian/Pa ic Islanders are one of the healthiest population groups, they still experience some health disparitie .

Health disparities between Asian/Pacific Islanders and other groups include the following:

- The mortality rate of Vietnamese women with cervical cancer is five times higher than that of white women.
- The incidences of newly diagnosed cases of hepatitis and tuberculosis are higher for Asian/Pacific Islanders than they are for the general population.
- The incidence of tuberculosis for Asian/Pacific Islanders is nearly five times higher than that of the total population.
- Asians have a greater risk of contracting hepatitis B, and more Asian people are infected with hepatitis B than are non-Asians. In most cases, Asians become infected with the hepatitis B virus when they are infants or young children. This occurs when infected mothers unknowingly pass on the virus to their babies at birth or when infants or young children are exposed to blood from another infected person with whom they live in close contact. When these children become adults, their immune systems can usually rid their bodies of the virus, and they usually recover.
- Despite certain health disparities, the infant mortality rate of Asian/Pacific Islanders is the lowest of any minority in the United States. This is a result of higher levels of education and better prenatal care than those of other minorities.
- Asian American women experienced the longest life expectancy (85.8 years) of any ethnic group in the United States.
- Asian Americans' leading causes of death in 2010 were cancer, heart disease, stroke, unintentional injuries (accidents), and diabetes. Death rates for these conditions are less than other racial/ethnic populations.

- Asian Americans are less likely to live in poverty (12.8%), more likely to be college graduates or hold graduate degrees (50%), and more likely to be employed in management, business, science, and arts occupations (48.5%) compared with the total U.S. population (15.9%, 28.5%, 36.0%, respectively) (www.cdc.gov).

American Indian & Alaska Native Populations

American Indians and Alaska Natives are people having origins in any of the original peoples of North and South America (including Central America), and who maintain tribal affiliation or community attachment. According to the U.S. Census Bureau in 2010, there were roughly 5.2 million American Indians and Alaska Natives living in the U.S., representing approximately 1.7 percent of the U.S. total population.

The projected U.S. population of American Indians and Alaska Natives for July 1, 2050 is estimated to reach 8.6 million.

Health disparities for American Indian and Alaska Natives:

- Higher mortality rates, with a life expectancy of five years less than the national average.
- Higher rates of tuberculosis, chronic liver disease and cirrhosis of the liver, accidents, diabetes, pneumonia, influenza, suicide, and homicide.
- Alcohol abuse, a very serious problem in Native American communities as a result of physiological and social factors related to the historic changes in their cultures.
- Large families with lower levels of education and income than the general population, which causes a low health status.

Like Asian/Pacific Islanders, however, Native populations have very low rates of infant mortality.

Immigrants

A **refugee** is a person who flees from one country or area to seek shelter or protection from danger in another area or country. An **immigrant** is a person who migrates from one country into another to find a permanent residence. An **alien** has no citizenship in the country in which he or she is residing. Aliens must eventually return to their original countries. An **illegal alien** is a person who flees from their homeland into another country without proper authorization.

A report published by the New York City Department of Health and Mental Hygiene, entitled *The Health of Immigrants in New York City*, found that immigrants or foreign-born New Yorkers were less likely than native New Yorkers or other American-born New Yorkers to have health insurance and therefore were less likely to have their blood pressure and cholesterol levels checked; experienced greater psychological distress; were less likely to have colon cancer screenings, pap tests, and mammograms; were less likely to receive immunization shots for flu and pneumonia; had higher rates of intimate-partner murder of females; had higher rates of tuberculosis; and had a higher rate of births for teen mothers than did U.S. citizens. As Dr. Thomas Frieden, former Commissioner of the New York City Department of Health and Mental Hygiene, explained, within the immigrant population "each subgroup has a distinct health profile." For example, the report indicates that Russian immigrants tend to be heavier smokers; Panamanian and Honduran immigrants are more likely to be obese; those from Ireland, Ghana, and Korea experience more episodes of binge drinking; and New Yorkers who were born in China had the highest mortality rate for liver cancer.

Although estimates vary significantly, some reports indicate that there are approximately 12 million people who are in the United States illegally. These illegal immigrants make up about 20 percent of the 46 million people who lack health insurance in the United States. In addition to those whose status is illegal and therefore cannot obtain health insurance, legal immigrants often have language barriers that prevent them from learning about health insurance coverage that might be available, understanding how to apply for health insurance, and even understanding how to maintain health insurance coverage. In addition, both language and cultural barriers present difficulties in communicating with doctors and other health care providers, including clearly understanding medical instructions. Such difficulties in communication can lead to serious health problems. To help mitigate the problems in health care caused by language and cultural barriers, many states have mandated that state applications for health care programs be offered in multiple languages. In addition, some states are hiring outreach workers and medically trained interpreters to reduce the problems that arise from miscommunication.

The United States has two large health care coverage programs available to immigrants: Medicaid and the State Children's Health Insurance Program (SCHIP).

- Medicaid is a government program that offers public assistance to people whose income and resources are insufficient to pay for health care.
- SCHIP is a program in which the federal government matches the funds of states to expand health insurance coverage to children.

Interventions to narrow the gap between immigrant and citizen health include:

- Government and public health agencies working to lower the barriers to health insurance enrollment
- Reducing language and cultural barriers
- Alleviating immigrants' concerns about participation in government health programs
- Providing education about the importance of obtaining health insurance and preventive health care

Health Disparities between Genders

Gender inequalities are differences that exist between men and women that empower one group to the detriment of the other. As in the social and political arenas, gender inequalities also exist in health status and access to health care.

An estimated 500,000 women die each year from cardiovascular disease, a higher rate than for men; however, there is a gap in the awareness of the need to identify and treat women for heart disease.

A study conducted by the Society for Women's Health Research indicated that a mere 3 percent of the total U.S. health budget was allocated to the study of gender differences. In fact, up until 1990, most clinical trials excluded women because researchers were concerned about women's hormonal changes and how those changes might influence the results of the studies.

Examples of gender health disparities include the following:

- Health disparities because of gender might be related, in part, to the exclusion of women from many clinical trials because of researchers' concerns about reproductive or menstrual issues.
- The life expectancy for women in the United States is 79.8, a little more than five years longer than the life expectancy for men, which is 74.4. Although women tend to live longer than men, they don't necessarily enjoy a better quality of life. Women who are 100 years of age or older outnumber men by a ratio of eight to one.

- Mortality rates from cancer are higher for men than for women.
- Sleep apnea, a potentially serious disorder that causes breathing to stop and start repeatedly during sleep, is more common in men than in women.
- Four times as many men commit suicide as women.
- Men tend to have fewer infection-fighting T-cells than women do.
- Even allowing for differences in size, with equal amounts of consumption of alcohol, women have higher blood alcohol contents than men do.
- Women who smoke cigarettes are more likely to develop lung cancer than are men who smoke the same amount of cigarettes.
- Women are more likely than men to suffer a second heart attack within one year of a first heart attack.
- The same drug can cause reactions and side effects that are different for women and men.
- Women are more likely than men are to acquire autoimmune diseases (diseases in which the body attacks its own tissues), such as lupus, rheumatoid arthritis, scleroderma, and multiple sclerosis.
- During unprotected intercourse with an infected partner, women are twice as likely as men to contract a sexually-transmitted disease, and 10 times more likely to contract HIV.
- Depression is two to three times more common in women than in men, partly because women's brains produce less of the hormone serotonin.
- After menopause, women lose more bone mass than men of similar age do.

Health Disparities and Food Insecurity

Minority populations seem to be the greatest affected when it comes to hunger and food insecurity in the United States. According to Feeding America, one in four African-American and Latino households is food insecure, compared to 11.4 percent of Caucasian households. Meanwhile, 32 percent of black children and nearly 35 percent of Latino children live in food-insecure households.

Health Disparities in the Name of Science

The United States government did something that was wrong—deeply, profoundly, morally wrong. It was an outrage to our commitment to integrity and equality for all our citizens . . . clearly racist.
—*President Clinton's apology for the Tuskegee Syphilis Experiment to the eight remaining survivors, May 16, 1997*

The Tuskegee Syphilis Experiment

Between 1932 and 1972, the U.S. Public Health Service (PHS) conducted an experiment on 399 African American men who were in the late stages of syphilis, a sexually-transmitted disease (STD). Researchers never told these men what disease they had or informed them about how serious the disease is. The intention of the study was to discover how syphilis affects African Americans compared with Caucasians. The theory was that syphilis made African Americans more susceptible to cardiovascular damage and that Caucasians were more susceptible to neurological complications from the disease. The men participating in the study were simply told that they were being treated for "bad blood;" the doctors conducting the study had no intention of treating them for or curing them of syphilis. Even when penicillin became commercially available in 1945, it was intentionally withheld from the Tuskegee men participating in the experiment. By the end of the experiment, 28 of the men had died directly from syphilis, 100 had died from related complications, 40 of their wives had been infected, and 19 of their children had been born with congenital syphilis.

The Tuskegee experiment continued despite both the passage of the Henderson Act of 1943, a public health law that required testing and treatment for sexually-transmitted diseases, and the World Health Organization's Declaration of Helsinki of 1964, which required "informed consent" from participants in experiments involving people.

Socioeconomic (SES) Disparities

> It is a crime to live in this rich nation and receive starvation wages.
> —*Dr. Martin Luther King, Jr., in a speech to sanitation workers, 1968*

The underlying causes of health disparities are imbalances in socioeconomic status. **Socioeconomic status** is the place or position in society that a person or family has based on social, economic, and educational factors. More than 60 percent of people who have no health insurance have low incomes or are members of low-income families. For obvious reasons, people who do not have health insurance receive less medical care, including preventive care, screening, and treatment, than do people who are covered by health insurance. In addition, even when those with no health insurance coverage do receive medical care, it often is of a poorer quality than the care of those who have health insurance.

Low socioeconomic status is linked to a wide range of health problems, including the following:

- Low birth weight
- Cardiovascular disease
- Hypertension
- Diabetes
- Cancer, with higher rates of mortality
- Arthritis
- A sedentary lifestyle, which can lead to other heath problems
- Inadequate consumption of fiber and fresh fruits and vegetables
- High rate of tobacco use, which is the greatest behavioral risk for premature mortality

Poverty creates conditions in which diseases frequently occur and spread, and are unlikely to be treated. More than one billion people throughout the world live on less than $1 per day.

Another health risk for people of low socioeconomic status is exposure to damaging substances in the environment. Such substances include lead, asbestos, carbon dioxide, and industrial wastes. These people are more likely than people of higher socioeconomic status to live and work in potentially harmful physical environments. In addition, poor neighborhoods are often located near highways, industrial areas, toxic waste sites, and other dangerous or unhealthy areas. As a result, people who live in such neighborhoods often have higher levels of lead in their blood, as well as higher rates of childhood asthma.

Did you know?

The homeless population in the U.S. includes people from all walks of life:

- More than 3.5 million people experience homelessness each year
- 35% of the homeless population are families with children, which is the fastest growing segment of the homeless population
- 23% are U.S. military veterans
- 25% are children under the age of 18
- 30% have experienced domestic violence
- 20-25% suffer from mental illness
- In urban communities, people experience homelessness for an average of eight months.
- The average minimum-wage worker must work 89 hours per week to be able to afford a two-bedroom apartment.

Why are people homeless today in America?

- Lack of affordable housing
- Lack of affordable medical care and health insurance
- Low wages and unemployment
- Cuts in social programs
- Other _____

Hurricane Katrina—Was this our first recent view into disparity?

As millions of people watched with horror the aftermath of Hurricane Katrina in 2005 on television, many wondered how such a human disaster could have happened in the United States. Many people alternated between outrage and grief as they saw endless footage of the failure of disaster relief services to materialize that we had assumed our government would provide. Appallingly, more than 1,000 citizens died because it took the government more than five days to distribute the necessary water, food, and medicine.

When one realizes who escaped the hurricane and its storm surge and who remained behind, it is impossible to ignore the shocking breadth of the gap between the rich and the poor. The reality is that poverty exists every day and in numerous places—it just isn't shown on TV as often as it was after Hurricane Katrina. For many of the more fortunate among us, the more than 37 million Americans living in poverty are unseen and unheard.

Of all the forms of inequality, injustice in health care is the most shocking and inhumane.
—*Dr. Martin Luther King, Jr.*

Health Care as a Health Disparity

The U.S. health care system is broken, but to fix the system successfully, we must first understand how, why, and where it is broken. The United States spends twice as much money as other developed countries do on health care, yet our health care system performs poorly in comparison. The bureaucracy of private insurance companies, including paperwork, consume approximately one-third of every health care dollar spent. Americans' average life expectancy of age 77 ranks 45th in the world, behind that of Bosnia and Jordan. In addition, the U.S. infant mortality rate is 6.37 per 1,000 live births, higher than that of most developed nations.

Many people in this country face major problems with their physical health. Cases of heart disease, diabetes, and obesity are increasing at alarming rates. For the first time in U.S. history, the life expectancy of children today is lower than their parents'.

The cost of health care causes a bankruptcy in the United States every 30 seconds.

A study called "Multinational Comparisons of Health Systems Data," found that, even though the U.S. spends the most of any country in the world on publicly and privately financed health insurance, Americans have the greatest number of years of life potentially lost as a result of circulatory diseases, respiratory diseases, and diabetes.

What differences create this disparity between the health care system of the United States and those of other developed countries?

Universal Health Care—The United States and South Africa are the only two industrialized countries in the world that do not have a national health care system that guarantees all citizens access to basic health benefits.

Major issues facing the U.S. health care system include:

- **Health disparities and discrimination:** People who are members of certain ethnic, racial, tribal, and religious minority groups may face health care discrimination and also experience language and cultural barriers.
- **Costs:** Approximately $2 trillion is spent each year on health care in the United States.
- **Access:** Some communities are underserved or not served at all, with no access to health care.
- **Quality of care and malpractice:** An estimated 44,000 to 98,000 people die every year because of medical errors.
- **Health promotion and disease prevention:** Greater emphasis needs to be placed on these areas of health care.

The United Nations has identified four criteria that are necessary for a successful health care system. These include the following:

Availability: It is essential that well functioning public health and health care facilities, services, medicines, and programs are available in sufficient quantity.

Accessibility: Health care facilities and services must be accessible to all people within a country. Accessibility includes four overlapping factors:

- Nondiscrimination
- Physical accessibility

- Affordability
- Information

Acceptability: All health care facilities and services must respect medical ethics, be culturally appropriate, be sensitive to the gender, lifestyle, and age requirements of patients, respect confidentiality, and be designed to improve the health status of patients.

Quality: Health facilities, medicines, and services must be scientifically and medically approved, appropriate, and of good quality.

If access to health care is considered a human right, who is considered human enough to have that right?

Access to health care is related to wealth, prestige, and education, but it is also related to power. If health is a human right, then it is a violation of human rights when national and international policies and practices interfere with a person's access to health care. It is unjust that mostly poor people do not have access to even a minimal level of health care.

A lack of health insurance coverage and gaps in such coverage is a problem that has long afflicted lower-income U.S. families. However, this is increasingly becoming a problem that affects many other Americans.

Many poor people are unable to visit doctors for relatively inexpensive preventive care, and thus, when health problems arise, they have no choice but to go to emergency rooms, where the cost of treatment is much higher. An estimated 2 million people in the United States go bankrupt every year as a result of medical debts that they cannot pay. A major study conducted by the Harvard Law School and Medical School indicated that many traditional middle-class families are just one major accident or illness away from economic hardship, bankruptcy, or poverty. According to the study, about half of all personal bankruptcies in the U.S. are a result, at least partially, of medical debts related to a major accident or illness; about 75 percent of those actually have health insurance at the time of the diagnosis of the illness or accident; and about 68 percent still have health insurance when they file for bankruptcy.

Poor health and a lack of health insurance is a vicious cycle: because those who are uninsured tend to be less healthy than the general population, they often cannot get better jobs, therefore they cannot afford health insurance; they then become even unhealthier, and when they become ill, they are likely to infect others in the community.

To improve the health of our population, greater emphasis must be placed on the promotion of health and the prevention of disease. The United States health care system currently does not encourage preventive services to the extent that it should. Surgeons who perform amputations on people with diabetes are paid huge sums of money, while dietitians who provide nutritional and dietary counseling are paid very little. Insurance companies spend large amounts of money for gastric bypass and other types of bariatric surgery (and enable overweight people to become obese so that they qualify for such types of surgery), instead of diverting that money to preventative care and nutrition education. With the focus in this country on quick fixes, such as prescription drugs, both doctors and consumers often overlook the vast amount of research showing that regular exercise, not smoking, and a healthful diet are the best ways to prevent illness and diseases; however, these simple steps do not generate large profits for the insurance industry. Investing in the prevention of diseases before they begin reduces the cost of health care later on.

The average American family spends between $10,000 and $12,000 every year for health insurance and other health care needs. If that family could instead invest this money in a typical mutual fund account, the family would have about $1 million in the account within 20 to 25 years.

Health care and health insurance *must* become a right, just as public education is, instead of a privilege only for the wealthy. The American ideal of life, liberty, and the pursuit of happiness can never be reached for working-class people, for the elderly, for many who already are ill, or for the poor, until every person in this country has access to adequate health care.

How Does American Health Care Compare To Taiwan?

They don't have to make the choice between a doctor's visit and paying their rent. In 1995, Taiwan chose William Hsiao, a professor of economics at the Harvard T.H. Chan School of Public Health, to lead a task force to design a new system. They adopted a single-payer system like that found in Canada.

Most hospitals in Taiwan remain privately owned, mostly nonprofit. Most physicians are still either salaried or self-employed in practices.

The health insurance Taiwan provides is comprehensive. Both inpatient and outpatient care are covered, as well as dental care, over-the-counter drugs and traditional Chinese medicine. Patients can choose from pretty much any provider or therapy. Wait times are short, and patients can go straight to specialty care without a referral. Premiums are paid for by the government, employers, and employees. The share paid by each depends on income, with the poor paying a much smaller percentage than the wealthy. Relative to the United States, Taiwan devotes less of its economy to health care. Taiwan has done a great job at treating many communicable diseases, but more chronic conditions are on the rise. These include cancer and cardiovascular and cerebrovascular disease.

Canadian Health Care System

The Canadian health care system addresses the problem of universal access to health care first, and then addresses its cost. In other words, each Canadian province must make sure that all its residents have access to medical care. The costs of this care are covered by a combination of public funds from provincial, federal, and corporate taxes, and from private funds. Canadian doctors are independent providers. As a result, Canadians spend much less on health care than Americans do, and there is a greater focus on prevention and primary care and less focus on specialized care.

National Health Services in Britain

The National Health Service (NHS) was established in 1948 to provide free health care for the citizens of the United Kingdom. The NHS is recognized as one of the best health care services in the world by the World Health Organization. The most important feature of the service for its founders was that it was free at the point of need. The NHS is funded through general taxes and is administered by the national Department of Health. The UK also has private health care providers, and people can opt to pay for private health care either through health insurance or when they use the services of these providers.

Cuba's Socialized Health Care

In 1976, the revised Cuban constitution stated that "Everyone has a right to health protection and care." In the movie *Sicko*, American filmmaker Michael Moore claims that the Cuban health care system is far superior to that of the United States. Cubans spend, on average, 1/25 the amount on health care as Americans do, and their health care is free for all. In *Sicko*, Michael Moore features a woman who formerly had a good job but was bankrupted by her medical bills and forced to live with her daughter. She paid $240 a month for cancer medication in the U.S. but gets the same pills in Cuba for 10 cents each. Michael Moore's production company also took along a number of Ground Zero responders who were ill to be treated in Cuba, because Cuban doctors had developed new techniques for treating lung cancer and other respiratory illnesses.

Members of a study seminar from the American Public Health Association have also visited Cuba, and they have seen both the problems and the strengths of the Cuban health care system. Cuba currently has more than 2,000 health care professionals who provide aid in 57 other countries. Cuba's uniquely resourceful health care system has continued to function well for decades, despite the U.S. embargo. Their focus on preventive care has resulted in greatly improved health indicators. For example, the incidence of infectious diseases that are preventable by vaccines is lower in Cuba than in any other nation at Cuba's level of economic development, because for many years, the rates of immunization have remained at between 99 and 100 percent of the target populations. Cuba has also implemented computerized surveillance at all provincial levels and is extending it to include municipalities and rural health care centers. This surveillance quickly identifies problems such as the spread of infectious diseases and changes in the distribution of chronic diseases. Such innovations may be instructive for countries, including the United States that lack efficient data-gathering and reporting systems for preventive services and efforts directed toward community-oriented primary care.

Cuba's difficulty in obtaining petroleum products motivated the import of more than a million bicycles, which have significantly reduced traffic congestion and pollution, in addition to improving the overall physical health of Cubans. Similarly, the scarcity of red meat in Cuba has led to relatively low rates of cholesterol and blood lipids. Despite the U.S. embargo on Cuba, which limits medicine and other supplies, all Cubans still receive free essential health care services.

Japan's Health Care

The Japanese have the longest life expectancy and the lowest infant mortality rate in the world yet spend half as much on health care as do Americans. Why? They have a cheap and universal health insurance system, called *kaihoken*, The Japanese people see doctors twice as often as Europeans and take more life-prolonging and life-enhancing drugs. They do not get pushed out of hospital beds prematurely; they stay in the hospital three times as long as the rich-world average, until treatment and recuperation is completely finished.

Swedish Health Care

Life expectancy in Sweden continues to rise—currently 79.1 years for men and 83.2 years for women. The Swedish health care system gives everyone who lives or works in Sweden equal access to heavily subsidized health care. The system is taxpayer-funded and largely decentralized. **Sweden introduced a health care guarantee in 2005.**

This means no patient should have to wait more than seven days for an appointment at a community health care center, 90 days for an appointment with a specialist, and 90 days for an operation or treatment, once it has been determined what care is needed.

References

Ayanian, J., Udvarhelyi, I., Gatsonis, C., Pashos, C., and Epstein, A. "Racial differences in the use of revascularization procedures after coronary angiography," *Journal of the American Medical Association*, 269 (1993): 642-646.

Association of American Medical Colleges. *Minority Graduates of U.S. Medical Schools: Trends, 1950-1998*, Washington, D.C.: Author, 2000.

Baldwin, D. "A model for describing low-income African American women's participation in breast and cervical cancer early detection and screening," *Advances in Nursing Science*, 19 (1996): 27-42.

Baldwin, D. and Nelms, T. "Difficult dialogues: Impact on nursing education curricula." *Journal of Professional Nursing*, 9(6) (1993), 3343-3346.

Bartlett, D. "The new health care consumer," *Journal of Health Care Finance*, 25 (1999): 44-51.

Brown, E. R., Pourat, N., and Wallace, S. P. "Undocumented residents make up small share of California's uninsured population," Los Angeles: UCLA Center for Health Policy Research, Fact Sheet, March 2007.

Byrne, M. "Uncovering racial bias in fundamental nursing textbooks: A critical hermeneutic analysis of the portrayal of African Americans," unpublished dissertation, Georgia State University: Atlanta, 2000.

Chen, M. S., and Hawks, B. L. "A debunking of the myth of healthy Asian Americans and Pacific Islanders," *American Journal of Health Promotion*, 9(4) (1995): 261-268.

Collins, K., Hall, A., and Neuhaus, C. *U.S. Minority health: A chartbook*. New York: The Commonwealth Fund, 1999.

Cooper-Patrick, L., Gallo, J., Gonzales, J, Vu., H., Powe, N., Nelson, C., and Ford, D. "Race, gender, and partnership in the patient-physician relationship," *JAMA*, 282(6) (1999): 583-589.

Cross, T., Bazron, B. J., Dennis, K. W., and Isaacs, M. R. *Towards a Culturally Competent System of Care*, vol. 1: Monograph on effective services for minority children who are severely emotionally disturbed. Washington, D.C.: CASSP Technical Assistance Center, Georgetown University Child Development Center, 1989.

DuBard, C. A., and Massing, M. W. "Trends in emergency Medicaid expenditures for recent and undocumented immigrants," *JAMA*, 297 (2007): 1085-1092.

Flegal, K. M., Carroll, M. D., Ogden C. L., and Johnson, C. L. "Prevalence and trends in obesity among U.S. adults, 1999-2000." *JAMA*, 288 (2002): 1723-1727.

Goldman, D. P., Smith, J. P., and Sood, N. "Immigrants and the cost of medical care," *Health Affairs*, (Millwood) 25 (2006): 1700-1711. http://content.nejm.org/cgi/ijlink?linkType=ABST&journalCode=healthaff&resid=25/6/1700

Grant, C. and Ladson-Billings, G. (eds.) *Dictionary of Multicultural Education*. Phoenix: Oryx Press, 1997.

Hannan, E., Van Ryn, M., Burke, J., Stone, D., Kumar, D., Arani, D., Pierce, W., Rafi, S., Sanborn, T., Sharma, S., Slater, J., and DeBuono, B. "Access to coronary artery bypass surgery by race/ethnicity and gender among patients who are appropriate for surgery," *Medical Care*, 37 (1999): 68-77.

Harris, L., Mungai, S., and Tierny, W. "Satisfaction with care in minority patients," in C. Hogue, M. Hargraves, & K. Collins (eds.), *Minority Health in America: Findings and Policy Implications from the Commonwealth Fund Minority Health Survey*, Baltimore: The John Hopkins University Press, 2000.

Herholz, H., Goff, D., Ramse, D., Chan, F., Ortiz, C., Labarthe, D., and Nichaman, M. "Women and Mexican Americans receive fewer cardiovascular drugs following myocardial infarction than men and non-Hispanic whites: The Corpus Christi Heart Project, 1988-1990," *Journal of Clinical Epidemiology*, 49(3) (1996): 279-287.

Hogue, C. "Eating well, exercising and avoiding smoking: Health promotion among men and women in minority populations," in C. Hogue, M. Hargraves, & K. Collins (eds.), *Minority Health in America: Findings and Policy Implications from the Commonwealth Fund Minority Health Survey*, Baltimore: The John Hopkins University Press, 2000.

Hogue, C. and Hargraves, M. "The commonwealth fund minority health survey of 1994: An overview," in C. Hogue, M. Hargraves, & K. Collins, *Minority Health in America: Findings and Policy Implications from the Commonwealth Fund Minority Health Survey*, Baltimore: The John Hopkins University Press, 2000.

Institute of Medicine. "Unequal treatment confronting racial and ethnic disparities in health care," *Institute of Medicine Report*, Washington, D.C.: National Academy Press, 2002.

Jones, J. H. *Bad Blood: The Tuskegee Syphilis Experiment*, expanded ed., New York: Free Press, 1993.

Jones, J. H. *Bad blood: The Tuskegee syphilis experiment*, New York: Macmillan, 1981.

Lancaster K. J., Watts, S. O., and Dixon, L. B. "Dietary intake and risk of coronary heart disease differ among ethnic subgroups of black Americans," *J Nutr.*, 136 (2006): 446-451.

Late, M. and Krisberg, K. "Hurricane Katrina creates public health crisis on U.S. Gulf Coast: Health, medical workers responding," *Nation's Health*, 35(8) (2005): 2005 American Public Health Association.

Leonard, T. "Exploring cultural, ethnic and racial diversity in baccalaureate nursing education programs," unpublished dissertation, Georgia State University: Atlanta, 2001.

McKinnon, J. "The black population in the United States: March 2000," *U.S. Census 2000 Bureau, Current Population Reports*, Series P20-541. Available at http://www.census.gov/prod/2003pubs/p20-541.pdf.

Mohanty, S. A., Woolhandler, S., Himmelstein, D. U., Pati, S., Carrasquillo, O., and Bor, D. H. "Health care expenditures of immigrants in the United States: A nationally representative analysis," *Am J Public Health*, 95 (2005): 1431-1438. http://content.nejm.org/cgi/ijlink?linkType=ABST&journalCode=ajph&resid=95/8/1431

National Institutes of Health. *Women of color health data book*. Office of the Director, Publication No.02-4247, Washington, D.C.: Author (2002).

New York City Department of Health and Mental Hygiene, *The Health of Immigrants in New York City*, New York: Author (June 2006).

Pear, R. "Lacking papers, citizens are cut from Medicaid," *New York Times*, March 12, 2007, A1.

Satcher, D. *U.S. Public Health Service, Department of Health and Human Services Before the House Commerce Committee*, Report from the Subcommittee on Health and Environment. Washington, D.C.: U.S. Public Health Service, Department of Health and Human Services (May 11, 2000).

Satel, S. "Race for the cure: Does racism make you sick?" *The New Republic*, 216(7) (1997): 12-13.

Smedley, B. D., Stith, A. Y., and Nelson, A. R. *Unequal treatment: Confronting racial and ethnic disparities in health care*. Institute of Medicine Report. Washington, D.C.: National Academy Press (2002).

Smith, D. B. *Health care divided: Race and healing a nation*. Ann Arbor: The University of Michigan Press, 1999.

Smith, L., "Are we reaching the health care consumer?" *Journal of Cultural Diversity*, 5(2) (1997): 48-52.

Society for Women's Health Research, www.womens-health.org.

U.S. Department of Health and Human Services, *A Century of Women's Health: 1900-2000*, Office of Women's Health, Washington, D.C.: Author, 2002.

U.S. Department of Commerce, Bureau of the Census, *Statistical Abstract of the United States*, Washington, D.C.: U.S. Government Printing Office, 2000.

U.S. Bureau of the Census, *Statistical Abstract of the United States*, Washington, D.C.: U.S. Government Printing Office, 2000.

U.S. Department of Health and Human Services, *Healthy People 2010: National Health Promotion and Disease Prevention Objectives* (Conference ed. in two vols.), Washington, D.C.: Author, 2000.

United States Kaiser Commission on Medicaid and the Uninsured, *Covering New Americans: A Review of Federal and State Policies Related to Immigrants' Eligibility and Access to Publicly Funded Health Insurance*. Shawn Fremstad and Laura Cox of the Center on Budget and Policy Priorities, November 2004.

Ward, E., Jemal, A., Cokkinides, V., Singh, G.K., Cardinez, C., Ghafoor, A., et al. "Cancer disparities by race/ethnicity and socioeconomic status," *CA Cancer J Clin.*, 54 (2004): 78-93.

Williams, D. R. "Race, socioeconomic status and health: The added effects of racism and discrimination," *Annals of the New York Academy of Sciences*, 896 (1999): 173-188.

www.hud user.org/publications/ povsoc/annual.assess.html, Report on the homeless in the U.S.

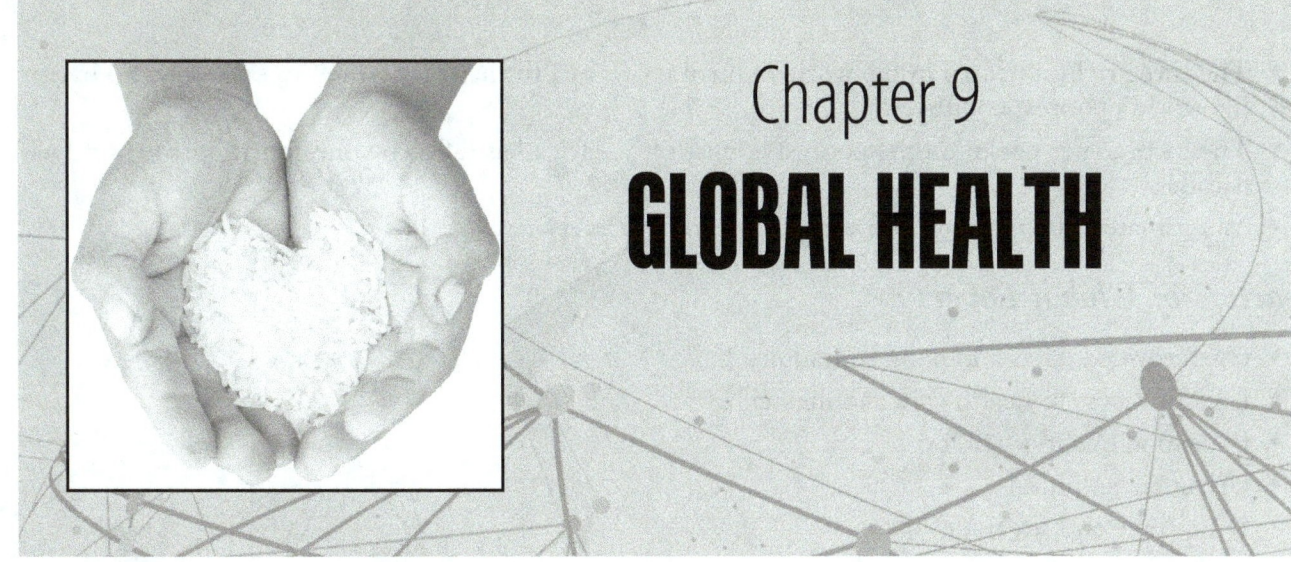

Chapter 9
GLOBAL HEALTH

The fact is that this generation—yours, my generation . . . we're the first generation that can look at poverty and disease, look across the ocean to Africa and say with a straight face, we can be the first to end this sort of stupid extreme poverty, where in the world of plenty, a child can die for lack of food in its belly. We have the cash, we have the drugs, and we have the science. Do we have the will to make poverty history?

—*Bono*

Many people, mostly in tropical countries of the Third World, die every day from preventable, curable diseases, such as malaria, tuberculosis, and AIDS. The toll on the world's population that is taken by infectious diseases is enormous: almost 33 million people around the world live with HIV/AIDS, an estimated 14 million people live with tuberculosis, and approximately 250 million people live with malaria. These people are dying because the drugs needed to treat these illnesses either do not exist or are unavailable. Despite incredible advances in medicine and health since the 1950s, many challenges remain, which should have already been solved.

Extreme Poverty and Hunger

Did You Know?

- About one-third of deaths—about 18 million people each year, or 50,000 each day—are from poverty-related causes.
- Every year, more than 10 million children die of hunger and preventable diseases—equal to more than 30,000 people per day and one every 3 seconds.
- More than 1 billion people survive on less than $1 a day, with almost half of the world's population of 2.8 billion surviving on less than $2 a day.
- About 600 million children live in conditions of absolute poverty.

- The three richest people in the world control more wealth than all 600 million people who live in the world's poorest countries.
- The income per person in the poorest countries in Africa has fallen by one-fourth in the past few decades.
- An estimated 800 million people go to bed hungry every day.

Factors of Global Poverty

- Overcrowded cities and poor sanitation
- Lack of access to health care and medicine
- Poor food quality
- Urban air pollution
- Drug trade and sex trade
- Lack of education

What is the relationship between poverty and disease?

Malaria, HIV/AIDS, and tuberculosis are among the diseases that disproportionately affect the world's poorest populations, which places a huge burden on the economies of developing countries.

Malaria

Malaria is a life-threatening parasitic disease that is transmitted by mosquitoes. The parasite infects a person from the bite of a female Anopheles mosquito, which requires blood to nurture her eggs. The infected person then transmits the disease to other people, who in turn transmit it to others. Malaria can kill people by destroying their red blood cells, causing anemia, and by clogging the capillaries that carry blood to the brain (cerebral malaria) or to other vital organs.

In Africa, malaria is both a disease of poverty and a cause of poverty. An African child dies every 30 seconds from malaria. Many children who do survive a case of severe malaria may suffer from learning impairments or brain damage. When the necessary drugs are not available or the parasites are resistant to the drugs, a malarial infection can progress rapidly to become life threatening. Displaced people, such as refugees, who live in makeshift housing, are especially vulnerable to malaria, because they are more likely to be bitten by mosquitoes, are often already ill with other infections, and lack access to adequate health care.

The human costs of malaria include the following:

- Loss of productivity
- Lost income associated with illness and death
- Human pain and suffering caused by the disease
- Negative consequences for children's schooling and social development both because of absenteeism and permanent neurological and other damage associated with severe cases of the disease.

Malaria is largely preventable and 100 percent treatable. Many poor people who do not have access to such basic preventable measures as bed nets treated with insecticide will die from the disease. Such a bed net costs only $5. One day's worth of spending on the military budget of the United States would provide all sleeping sites in Africa with five years of bed-net coverage, which would eradicate a disease that kills millions every year.

Priority Actions

- Provide universal access to insecticide-treated bed nets.
- Spray indoor surfaces with long-lasting insecticides.
- Provide funding for more effective drugs.

Tuberculosis

Tuberculosis (TB) is a contagious respiratory disease that is spread through the air. When people infected with TB cough, sneeze, talk, or spit, they release TB bacilli into the air. Another person need only inhale a small number of these bacilli to become infected. Symptoms of TB include fever, weight loss, night sweats, and the coughing up of blood. However, people who are infected with TB bacilli do not necessarily experience symptoms of the disease right away. The body's immune system can hide the TB bacilli, which are protected by a thick waxy coat, and they can lie dormant for years. When a person's immune system becomes weakened, the chances of the person becoming ill from the TB bacilli increase.

An especially dangerous form of TB is multidrug-resistant TB (MDR-TB), which is the disease caused by TB bacilli that is resistant to anti-TB drugs. MDR-TB is caused by inconsistent or partial treatment for the disease, for example, by patients who do not take all their prescribed medicines regularly and for the necessary period because they feel better; because doctors or other health workers administer the wrong treatment regimens; or because the drug supply is unreliable. The fatality rate for MDR-TB is six times higher than the rate for non-MDR-TB.

Approximately one-third of the world's population is currently infected with TB bacilli. Many people likely would be shocked and saddened to learn that one of the leading causes of death throughout the world is a disease for which treatment has been available since the mid-twentieth century with rates of recovery of about 95 percent.

Priority Actions

- Treat active TB cases quickly.
- Manage multidrug resistant TB with new drugs and drug combinations.
- Provide free access for testing and treatment.
- Develop a low-cost vaccine against pulmonary TB.

STDs

Every year in the United States, 4 million teenagers contract an STD.

Why Young People Have High Risk of STDs:

- Feeling of invulnerability
- Multiple sex partners
- Not using condoms
- Drugs and alcohol

Chlamydia is a curable infection caused by the bacteria *Chlamydia trachomatis.*

Transmission

- Chlamydia can be transmitted during vaginal, anal, and oral sex. Using latex condoms consistently and correctly—from the very beginning of sexual contact until there is no longer skin contact—reduces the risk of transmission of chlamydia.

Symptoms

- Most women and some men do *not* experience symptoms. If symptoms do occur, they usually appear within one to three weeks after infection.
- In women, if left untreated, chlamydia can cause complications such as pelvic inflammatory disease (PID) and infertility.
- In men, untreated chlamydia can cause burning and discharge during urination, inflammation of scrotal skin, and testicular swelling.

Gonorrhea is a curable infection caused by the bacteria *Neisseria gonorrhoea.*

Transmission

- Gonorrhea is transmitted during vaginal, anal, and oral sex.

Symptoms

- Many men infected with gonorrhea exhibit symptoms, whereas most women are asymptomatic. Even when women do have symptoms, they can be mistaken for a bladder infection or other vaginal infection.
- In men, symptoms usually appear within two to nine days after infection, with possible thick yellow or white pus emerging from the penis or a burning sensation.
- In women, if left untreated, gonorrhea can cause complications such as PID and infertility.
- In both genders, if left untreated, gonorrhea can lead to arthritis in joints and can attack the heart muscle, skin, and brain.

Pelvic inflammatory disease (PID) is a serious infection in the upper genital tract/reproductive organs (uterus, fallopian tubes, and ovaries) of a female. PID can be sexually transmitted or naturally occurring. It can lead to infertility in women or life-threatening complications. Women between ages 15 and 25 have the highest incidence of PID. In the United States, PID is the leading cause of infertility in women.

Transmission

- Chlamydia and gonorrhea are the most common causes of PID.
- If you have an infection in the genital tract and do not get treated right away, it can cause PID.
- The infection spreads from the cervix into the uterus, fallopian tubes, and ovaries. It can take anywhere from several days to several months after being infected to develop PID.

Symptoms

- It is possible for a woman to have PID and be asymptomatic (without symptoms), or have symptoms too mild to notice, for an unknown period of time.
- Dull pain or tenderness in the lower abdomen
- Burning or pain when you urinate
- Nausea and vomiting
- Bleeding between menstrual periods
- Increased or changed vaginal discharge
- Pain during sex
- Fever and chills

- PID can also be misdiagnosed as appendicitis, ectopic pregnancy, ruptured ovarian cysts, or other problems.

Genital HPV is caused by human papillomavirus (HPV). Human papillomavirus is the name of a group of viruses that includes more than 100 different strains or types.

Some of these viruses are called "high-risk" types, and may cause abnormal Pap tests. They may also lead to cancer of the cervix, vulva, vagina, anus, or penis. Others are called "low-risk" types, and they may cause mild Pap test abnormalities or genital warts. Genital warts are single or multiple growths or bumps that appear in the genital area, and sometimes are cauliflower shaped.

Approximately 20 million people are currently infected with HPV. At least 50 percent of sexually active men and women acquire genital HPV infection at some point in their lives. By age 50, at least 80 percent of women will have acquired genital HPV infection. About 6.2 million Americans get a new genital HPV infection each year.

Transmission

- The types of HPV that infect the genital area are spread primarily through genital contact.

Symptoms

- Most HPV infections have no signs or symptoms; therefore, most infected persons are unaware they are infected, yet they can transmit the virus to a sex partner.

Chancroid is a curable infection caused by bacteria called *Haemophilus Ducrey*. Chancroid causes ulcers or sores, usually of the genitals. Swollen, painful lymph glands in the groin area are often associated with chancroid.

Transmission

- Left untreated, chancroid may make the transmission of HIV easier. Chancroid is transmitted in two ways:
- Sexual transmission through skin-to-skin contact with an open sore.
- Nonsexual transmission when contact is made with the pus-like fluid from the ulcer.

Symptoms

- Soft painful sores or a smelly discharge. A person is considered to be infectious (able to pass the bacteria to others) when ulcers or sores are present. This means that as long as there are chancroid sores on the body, the person can spread the infection.

Crabs (also known as pubic lice) are small parasites that feed on human blood. Crabs are not the same as head and body lice. Crabs are usually found on the pubic hair, but can be also be found on other parts of the body where a person has coarse hair (such as armpits, eyelashes, and facial hair). Crabs rarely infest head hair.

Transmission

- Anyone can get crabs. Having crabs does not mean a person is unclean or dirty.
- A person can get crabs during sexual contact with a person who has crabs. During the close physical contact, the crabs can move from the pubic hair of one person to the pubic hair of another. Crabs can be sexually transmitted even if there is no penetration or exchange of body fluids.
- Once off a human host, crabs can live for 24 hours, making it possible to get crabs during contact with infested bedding or clothing.

Symptoms

- The most noticeable symptom of crabs is itching. The itching usually starts about five days after a person gets crabs.

Scabies is a curable skin disease caused by the parasite *Sarcoptes scabiei*.

Transmission

- Scabies is transmitted through close physical contact with a person who is infected or prolonged contact with infested linens, furniture, or clothing.

Symptoms

- The most common symptom is itching, which usually occurs within four to six weeks after infection.
- A person is considered infectious from the time of infestation until treatment is successfully completed.

Syphilis is a sexually transmitted disease caused by the bacterium *Treponema pallidum*. Pregnant women with the disease can pass it to babies. Genital sores (chancres) caused by syphilis make it easier to sexually transmit and acquire HIV infection. There is an estimated two- to five-fold increased risk of acquiring HIV infection when syphilis is present.

Transmission

- Syphilis is passed from person to person through direct contact with a syphilis sore.
- Sores occur mainly on the lips, mouth, external genitals, vagina, anus, or in the rectum.
- Transmission of the organism occurs during vaginal, anal, or oral sex.
- Syphilis cannot be spread through contact with toilet seats, doorknobs, swimming pools, hot tubs, bathtubs, shared clothing, or eating utensils.

Primary Stage

- The primary stage of syphilis is usually marked by the appearance of a single sore (called a chancre), but there may be multiple sores.
- The time between infection with syphilis and the start of the first symptom can range from 10 to 90 days (average 21 days).
- The chancre is usually firm, round, small, and painless. It appears at the spot where syphilis entered the body.
- The chancre lasts three to six weeks, and it heals without treatment. However, if adequate treatment is not administered, the infection progresses to the secondary stage.

Secondary Stage

- This stage typically starts with the development of a rash on one or more areas of the body. The rash usually does not cause itching.
- The characteristic rash of secondary syphilis may appear as rough, red, or reddish brown spots both on the palms of the hands and the bottoms of the feet.
- In addition to rashes, symptoms of secondary syphilis may include fever, swollen lymph glands, sore throat, patchy hair loss, headaches, weight loss, muscle aches, and fatigue.

Late Stage

- The latent (hidden) stage of syphilis begins when secondary symptoms disappear.
- In the late stages of syphilis, it may subsequently damage the internal organs, including the brain, nerves, eyes, heart, blood vessels, liver, bones, and joints.
- Signs and symptoms of the late stage of syphilis include difficulty coordinating muscle movements, paralysis, numbness, gradual blindness, and dementia. This damage may be serious enough to cause death.

Bacterial vaginosis (BV) is a condition in women in which the normal balance of bacteria in the vagina is disrupted and replaced by an overgrowth of certain bacteria. BV is the most common vaginal infection in women of childbearing age. In the United States, as many as 16 percent of pregnant women have BV.

Symptoms

- Discharge, odor, pain, itching, or burning.
- Discharge, if present, is usually white or gray; it can be thin.
- Some women with BV report no signs or symptoms at all.

Some activities or behaviors can upset the normal balance of bacteria in the vagina and put women at increased risk, including:

- Having a new sex partner or multiple sex partners.
- Douching.
- Using an intrauterine device (IUD) for contraception.

In most cases, BV causes no complications. However, some serious risks exist from having BV, including:

- Can increase a woman's susceptibility to HIV infection if she is exposed to the HIV virus.
- Increases the chances that an HIV-infected woman can pass HIV to her sex partner.
- Has been associated with an increase in the development of pelvic inflammatory disease (PID) following surgical procedures such as a hysterectomy or an abortion.
- While pregnant may put a woman at increased risk for some complications of pregnancy.
- Can increase a woman's susceptibility to other STDs, such as chlamydia and gonorrhea.

Genital herpes is an infection of the genitals, buttocks, or anal area caused by herpes simplex virus (HSV). According to the Centers for Disease Control and Prevention, one out of five American teenagers and adults is infected with HSV type 2. Women are more commonly infected than men.

There are two types of HSV:

- HSV type 1 most commonly infects the mouth and lips, causing sores known as fever blisters or cold sores. It is also an important cause of sores to the genitals.
- HSV type 2 is the usual cause of genital herpes, but it also can infect the mouth.

Transmission

- Most people get genital herpes by having sex with someone who is shedding the herpes virus either during an outbreak or during a period with no symptoms.
- Herpes can be transmitted through close contact other than sexual intercourse, through oral sex or close skin-to-skin contact, for example.
- In most people, the virus can become active and cause outbreaks several times a year. This is called a recurrence, and infected people can have symptoms.
- HSV remains in certain nerve cells of your body for life. When the virus is triggered to be active, it travels along the nerves to your skin. There, it makes more viruses and sometimes new sores near the site of the first outbreak.
- Do not have oral or genital contact in the presence of any symptoms or findings of oral herpes.

Symptoms (Outbreaks)

- Symptoms might include tingling or sores near the area where the virus has entered the body, such as on the genital or rectal area, on buttocks or thighs, or occasionally on other parts of the body where the virus has entered through broken skin.

- Small red bumps appear first, develop into small blisters, and then become itchy, painful sores that might develop a crust and will heal without leaving a scar.
- Other symptoms are fever, headache, muscle aches, painful or difficult urination, vaginal discharge, and swollen glands in the groin area.
- Sometimes, the virus can become active but not cause any visible sores or any symptoms. During these times, small amounts of the virus may be shed at or near places of the first infection, in fluids from the mouth, penis, or vagina, or from barely noticeable sores. This is called asymptomatic (without symptoms) shedding. Even though you are not aware of the shedding, you can infect a sexual partner during this time. Asymptomatic shedding is an important factor in the spread of herpes.

Birth Control

Under the right circumstances, sexual relations can be a wonderful part of a relationship. Sexual relations can provide a couple with intimacy, a unique bond, and emotional fulfillment. Engaging in a sexual relationship at the wrong time, with the wrong person, or under the wrong circumstances can cause you a lot of grief. No matter what your age, some issues must be considered before becoming sexually intimate with someone. *No* method of birth control prevents pregnancy all of the time. Birth control methods can fail, but you can greatly increase a method's success rate by using it correctly all of the time. The only way to be sure you never get pregnant is to not have sex (abstinence).

The birth control method you choose should take into account:

- Your overall health.
- How often you have sex.
- Number of sexual partners you have.
- If you want to have children.
- How well each method works (or is effective) in preventing pregnancy.
- Any potential side effects.
- Your comfort level with using the method.

Following is a list of birth control methods with estimates of effectiveness, or how well they work in preventing pregnancy when used correctly, for each method:

Continuous abstinence—This means not having sexual intercourse (vaginal, anal, or oral intercourse) at any time. It is the only sure way to prevent pregnancy and protect against HIV and other STDs. This method is 100 percent effective in preventing pregnancy and STDs.

The male condom—Condoms are called barrier methods of birth control because they put up a block, or barrier, which keeps the sperm from reaching the egg. Only latex or polyurethane (because some people are allergic to latex) condoms are proven to help protect against STDs, including HIV. "Natural" or "lambskin" condoms are not recommended for STD prevention because they have tiny pores that may allow for the passage of viruses like HIV, hepatitis B, and herpes. Male condoms are 84 to 98 percent effective at preventing pregnancy.

Oral contraceptives—Also called "the pill," oral contraceptives contain the hormones estrogen and progestin. They are taken daily to block the release of eggs from the ovaries. They do not protect against STDs or HIV. Oral contraceptives lighten the flow of your period and can reduce the risk of pelvic inflammatory disease (PID), ovarian cancer, benign ovarian cysts, endometrial cancer, and iron deficiency anemia. The pill is 95 to 99.9 percent effective in preventing pregnancy.

Side Effects
- Oral contraceptives increase the risk of heart disease, including high blood pressure, blood clots, and blockage of the arteries, especially if you smoke.
- Some antibiotics may reduce the effectiveness of the pill. Talk to your doctor or nurse about a back-up method of birth control if she or he prescribes antibiotics.

The female condom—Worn by the woman, this barrier method keeps sperm from getting into her body. It is made of polyurethane, is packaged with a lubricant, and may protect against STDs, including HIV. It can be inserted up to 24 hours prior to sexual intercourse. Female condoms are 79 to 95 percent effective at preventing pregnancy.

Side Effects
- Some people may experience irritation as a result of wearing the condom, but the risk is not as great as with latex condoms.
- Trouble inserting the condom.
- In some cases, the condom may shift or slip into the vagina during sex, making the condom somewhat ineffective.
- Some people may also find that the outer ring makes sex uncomfortable, whereas others find that the outer ring is useful in stimulating the clitoris.
- Female condoms are more expensive than male condoms.

Emergency contraceptives are methods of *preventing* pregnancy *after* unprotected sexual intercourse. Emergency contraception is often called "the morning after pill," but this is misleading because emergency contraception can be used *before* the morning after or up to five days after. Emergency contraceptives *do not* protect against sexually transmitted infections. Emergency contraception can be used when a condom breaks, after a sexual assault, or any time unprotected sexual intercourse occurs.

Emergency contraceptives include: Emergency contraceptive pills (ECPs) are sometimes wrongly called "the morning after pill." This is wrong because ECPs are never taken as one pill, the "morning after." They are taken in two doses, 12 hours apart. They work best if taken within 72 hours of unprotected vaginal intercourse. ECPs contain higher doses of hormones than those contained in birth control pills.
Emergency contraception keeps a woman from getting pregnant by stopping:

- Ovulation, or stopping the ovaries from releasing eggs that can be fertilized.
- Fertilization, or stopping the egg from being fertilized by the sperm.
- Implantation, or stopping a fertilized egg from attaching itself to the wall of the uterus.

Planned Parenthood health center: 1-800-230-PLAN or 1-800-230-7526

Global AIDS

Did You Know?

According to the Centers for Disease Control and Prevention:

- More than 1.1 million people in the United States are living with HIV infection, and almost 1 in 5 (18.1%) are unaware of their infection.
- Gay, bisexual, and other men who have sex with men (MSM),[1] particularly young black/African American MSM, are most seriously affected by HIV.
- By race, African Americans face the most severe burden of HIV.
- In Africa, 6,500 people die of AIDS every day, and another 9,500 contract the HIV virus, 1,400 of which are newborns who are infected during childbirth or by their mothers' milk.
- So far, more than 11 million African children have lost at least one parent to HIV/AIDS.
- About 5 people die every minute from AIDS.
- Almost 3 million children are living with AIDS, and more than 4 million have died of AIDS since the epidemic began.
- About 1 in every 100 people worldwide is HIV positive, and one-third of these are between the ages of 15 and 24.

HIV (human immunodeficiency virus) is the virus that causes AIDS. This virus can be transmitted from one person to another when infected blood, semen, or vaginal secretions come in contact with an uninfected person's broken skin or mucous membranes. Pregnant women who are infected with HIV can pass it on to their babies during pregnancy or delivery, and mothers of newborns can transmit the virus to their babies through breastfeeding. The human immunodeficiency virus that causes AIDS can be transmitted via blood, breast milk, and by semen during sex, but can be kept in check with cocktails of drugs known as antiretroviral treatment or therapy.

The most common ways in which HIV spreads are through sexual contact, the sharing of needles for illicit drug use, and transmission from infected mothers to babies. The transmission of HIV through sexual contact can occur from men to men, men to women, women to men, and women to women through vaginal, anal, and oral sex. The best way to prevent sexual transmission of HIV is abstinence from sexual contact until both partners in a monogamous relationship are certain that they are not infected with HIV. Because an HIV antibody test can take up to 6 months to indicate a positive result, both partners should test negative 6 months after their last potential exposure to HIV before having sexual relations. Aside from abstinence, the use of latex condoms is the next-best method of preventing the spread of HIV through sexual contact.

Symptoms of HIV first became noticed in 1981 among homosexual men in Los Angeles and New York. These men had an unusual type of pneumonia and rare skin tumors called Kaposi's sarcoma. They also had dangerously low levels of T cells in their blood. T cells are an important part of the immune system and help the body fight infections. In 1985, a blood test became available to measure antibodies to HIV that are the body's immune response to the HIV virus. Currently, tests are available to detect these same antibodies in saliva and urine; some can provide results within 20 minutes of testing.

HIV is a virus that infects the body's cells and makes new copies of itself within those cells. The virus can also damage human cells, which is one of the ways in which it can cause a person to become ill. As time goes on, a person who is infected with HIV is likely to become ill more and more often. At some point, usually several years after they became infected, they are afflicted with one of a variety of severe illnesses, which ultimately will kill them. A person does not die of AIDS, but rather from complications of common diseases, such as a cold, the flu, or pneumonia, because at that stage of HIV infection, the body's immune system has very little defense against any kind of infection.

Approximately 42 million people around the world are now living with HIV and AIDS, which respects no borders, no economic class, no gender, and no age. The fact that health care services in poor countries lack doctors and nurses, combined with the high price of drugs, means that the vast majority of poor people have no access to treatment. More than 20 million people have died of complications from AIDS since the disease was first identified in 1981, and about 3 million people currently die from such complications every year.

However, many countries, including Brazil, Uganda, and Thailand, have been successful in reducing rates of HIV infection. Politicians are increasingly making a commitment to fight the spread of the disease in their countries, and medicines to treat it are becoming increasingly available in poor countries. Still, the incidence of AIDS remains incredibly high in Africa. The disease is now spreading most quickly in Eastern Europe and Asia, which includes about 60 percent of the world's population.

HIV/AIDS in the United States—from a death sentence to a chronic illness.

In the United States, HIV/AIDS began in the early 1980s as an epidemic primarily viewed as affecting gay, white men. The epidemic has since changed in that it disproportionately affects African Americans. According to the Centers for Disease Control and Prevention (CDC), African Americans currently account for more than half of all HIV/AIDS cases in the U.S., and HIV/AIDS is now the leading cause of death among African American women between the ages of 25 and 34. African American women in the United States are diagnosed with HIV/AIDS at a rate 23 times higher than white women, while African American men are diagnosed at a rate 7 times higher than white men. The estimated incidence of HIV has remained stable overall in recent years, at about 50,000 new HIV infections per year. Approximately 636,000 people in the United States with an AIDS diagnosis have died since the epidemic began.

Women are at a disproportionately higher risk for contracting HIV for the following reasons:

- Poverty
- Sexual abuse
- Married men secretly also having sex with other men
- Lack of female-controlled HIV prevention methods
- Disparities in access to health care
- Imbalances of power
- Threats of sexual violence (rape, incest, abuse), which deter women from trying to persuade men to practice safer sex or to resist unprotected sex.

Health officials who have been tracking the disproportionate rates of AIDS-related deaths among minorities over the past several years suggest that those rates are a result of such factors as a failure to identify those who are infected and provide them with treatment, a failure to persuade those who are being treated to continue with the treatment, and the strong stigma that AIDS has in many minority communities.

Children

More than half of all new HIV infections in the United States are now occurring in young people under the age of 25. Every minute of every day, a child under the age of 15 becomes infected with HIV. In most of these cases, the virus is transmitted by an HIV-infected mother to her fetus, during delivery, or through breastfeeding after birth. An estimated 90 percent of the more than 5 million children in the

U.S. who are HIV-infected were born in Africa. The other most common causes of HIV infection in children include contaminated blood products or syringes and sexual abuse.

Prevention of maternal and childhood HIV:

- HIV prevention education and family planning for all women of childbearing age.
- Counseling, testing, and access to antiretroviral treatment for all those infected.
- Education on how to avoid unintended pregnancy.
- Steps to reduce the risk of transmission during and after pregnancy.
- Direct confrontation of child sexual abuse.
- Education and access to confidential, low-cost, and youth-friendly contraceptive services for sexually active youths to reduce teenage pregnancies and help them protect themselves from sexually-transmitted diseases and HIV infection.

Abstinence-Only Education vs. Age Appropriate Health Education

A national study completed in 2007 concluded that abstinence-only sex education does not prevent teenagers from having sex, nor does it have any affect on the likelihood that when they do have sex, they will use a condom. In contrast, responsible sex-education programs have been shown to have such positive results as teenagers delaying having sex, reducing the frequency of sexual encounters, and increasing contraceptive use.

The United States has unacceptably high rates of teenage pregnancies, sexually-transmitted diseases (STDs), and HIV/AIDS infections. To address this problem, we must support age-appropriate and medically accurate health-education programs that promote abstinence *and* provide adolescents with the information that they need to protect themselves if they do choose to be sexually active. Research indicates that honest, medically accurate sex education works, while abstinence-only programs do not. Many abstinence-only programs include false and misleading information, which teenagers often pick up on.

Harm Reduction

Harm-reduction programs allow intravenous drug users to exchange dirty needles for sanitary needles. The thinking behind harm reduction programs is that if a clean supply of needles is available to intravenous drug users, they will be less likely to share needles with other users, thereby reducing the risk of infecting themselves and others with HIV.

HIV Medication

HIV is a type of virus called a retrovirus, and drugs that disrupt the action of HIV are called antiretrovirals. These have proven to be very effective in treating people with AIDS, but they cannot cure AIDS. HAART is a form of treatment that includes antiretroviral drugs and significantly delays the progression from HIV to AIDS. HAART has been available in wealthy countries since 1996, but in less-wealthy and poor countries, very few people who are HIV-positive can afford this treatment.

Access to treatment is one of the major concerns of people who are infected with HIV/AIDS, most of whom cannot afford the necessary health care and antiretrovirals. Access to drugs, to some degree, also depends upon people being aware of their HIV status, knowledgeable about treatment, and empowered to seek such treatment.

The Role of Big Pharmaceutical Companies

To some extent, HIV/AIDS is a disease of poverty. When poverty contributes to the spread of a disease or causes a disease in a community, large pharmaceutical companies benefit by holding power and influence, especially in poorer countries. One of the major reasons for unnecessary deaths worldwide is that people simply cannot afford life-saving medication that does exist. Sadly, millions of people die from preventable or curable diseases every week.

Multinational pharmaceutical companies often ignore certain diseases in under-developed countries because there is no profit to be made there. Instead, these companies concentrate on producing more drugs that lead to high profits, such as new medications for headaches and erectile dysfunction.

A documentary entitled *Dying for Drugs* reveals how one of the world's largest pharmaceutical companies experimented on children in Africa without their parents' knowledge or consent. The film also showed how a drug company attempted to silence a prominent expert in Canada who had doubts about the efficacy or safety of a particular drug that the company manufactured. In South Korea, the documentary followed the attempts of desperately ill patients to convince a leading pharmaceutical company to provide them with life-saving drugs at a price that they could afford. Finally, the film showed a 12-year-old Honduran child dying from AIDS and people trying to help him by smuggling the drugs that he needed across the Guatemalan border, breaking the law in the process, simply to obtain the drugs at affordable prices. The child died as the documentary crew was filming the desperate smuggling.

In India, patent laws allow the production of cheap generic drugs. The Chemical, Industrial & Pharmaceutical Laboratories (CIPLA) is a large Indian pharmaceutical company best-known outside of India for its manufacture and distribution of a low-cost antiretroviral for HIV-positive people in developing countries, even though the company took a loss in profit. Company representatives said that CIPLA made profits from other drugs, and that this undertaking was about more than a matter of profit and loss. However, the Indian government has been pressured about its patent laws by wealthy countries for some time. When CIPLA offered to provide a cocktail of antiretroviral drugs for AIDS at the price of $350 a year, compared to the $10,000 charged by multinational pharmaceutical companies, this sent shockwaves to both large pharmaceutical companies and to poor countries. Poor countries realized that there actually was a more affordable way to deal with the HIV/AIDS health crisis, which afflicted them the most, while the large multinational drug companies saw their monopoly prices not only exposed, but also threatened.

As a result of the bad publicity generated by this incident, many large pharmaceutical companies began to offer AIDS antiretrovirals and other drugs at cheaper prices and even donated large amounts of money to global HIV/AIDS initiatives. Former President Clinton's HIV/AIDS Initiative (CHAI) has been working to lower the prices that people in developing countries have to pay for AIDS antiretrovirals. CHAI has become a major force in helping poor countries to negotiate prices with pharmaceutical companies and to obtain faster AIDS tests.

Priority actions to reduce the spread of HIV/AIDS include the following:

- Promote 100% condom use and education, especially among populations at high risk.
- Treat other sexually-transmitted diseases that increase the risk of HIV infection.
- Provide antiretroviral medications, especially for pregnant women.
- Offer harm-reduction programs (e.g., needle exchanges) for intravenous drug users.
- Offer voluntary counseling and testing for HIV.
- Combat the stigma and discrimination surrounding HIV and AIDS.

Maternal and Child Health

Maternal and child health is one of the major subfields of public health. Child health professionals pay special attention to children in their first 5 years of life, who are most vulnerable among children to illnesses and death.

It is a disgrace that so many children die of diseases that are easily preventable. The silent killers are poverty, hunger, and easily-preventable diseases and illnesses.

More than 25,000 children die every day around the world, which is equivalent to:

- 1 child dying every 3.5 seconds.
- 17-18 children dying every minute.
- A 2004 Asian Tsunami occurring almost every 1.5 weeks.
- More than 9 million children dying every year.
- Approximately 70 million children dying between 2000 and 2007.

Child Deaths Under Age 5 in 2007.

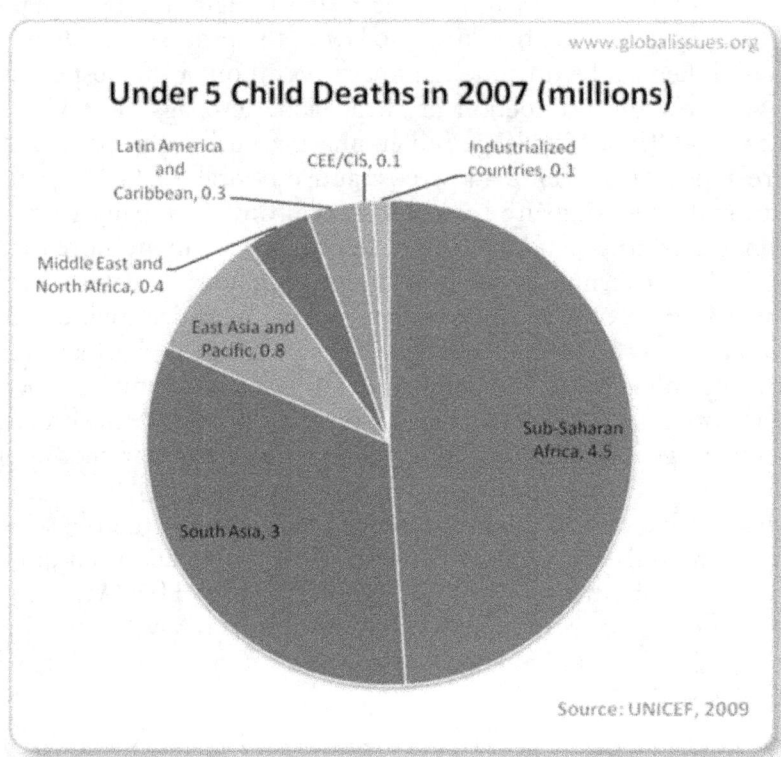

Goal: Reduce Child Mortality

Leading Causes of Death of Children Globally:

- Malnutrition
- Pneumonia
- Diarrhea
- Measles
- Malaria

Factors for Deaths of Children Globally:

- **Poverty** is the root cause of high rates of child mortality and morbidity. A lack of sanitation pollutes the water that children drink, and poor nutrition makes them vulnerable to illnesses and diarrhea, which, if left untreated, can cause dehydration and further reduce a child's body weight and resistance to disease.

- **Armed Conflicts:** As wars proliferate, hundreds of thousands of children are caught up in conflicts by being forced to become soldiers; being refugees; and suffering sexual violence, abuse, and exploitation. Even when children caught in conflicts are not killed or injured, they can be orphaned, abducted, raped, and left with emotional scars and trauma from direct exposure to violence or from dislocation and the loss of family members. Even when these conflicts end, there is still the danger of abandoned explosives and weapons, and landmines, which kill and maim thousands of children every year.

- **HIV/AIDS** is the leading cause of death in the world for people aged 15 to 49. Every day, approximately 1,800 children, most of them newborns, become infected with HIV. Without HIV medication, about 45 percent of HIV-infected children die before they reach the age of 2. Often, the consumption of food in an AIDS-affected household declines, especially when the person suffering from AIDS is an adult who had previously helped to support the family. This leaves children at a higher risk for malnutrition and under-nutrition. Many children whose families are affected by HIV/AIDS, especially girls, are forced to drop out of school so they can work or care for their families.

- **Trafficking and Child Labor:** An estimated 1.2 million children throughout the world are bought and sold every year, and about 2 million children, the majority of them girls, are exploited in the commercial sex industry. Some children are bought and forced to work in sweatshops or as farm workers harvesting coffee. Currently, approximately 180 million children are engaged in some form of child labor.

   The trafficking of children often involves the exploitation of their parents' extreme poverty. Parents may sell children to traffickers to pay off debts or to supplement their income; sometimes they are deceived about the prospects of education, training, and a better life than they can provide for their children. In West Africa, children who are sold have often lost one or both parents to AIDS.

- **Malnutrition and Under-Nutrition.** The World Health Organization (WHO) cites under-nutrition as the largest single contributor to the premature deaths of children. Infants who weigh less than 5.5 pounds at birth are at greater risk for diseases and death than are infants with a normal birth weight, which is about 8.5 pounds. Under-nutrition is an underlying cause of an estimated 53 percent of all deaths of children younger than age 5.

The first step in preventing the deaths of children is to make sure that every child is well nourished and has safe and adequate food and water.

Pneumonia in children under 5 years of age is the leading cause of childhood mortality worldwide. More than 2 million children die from pneumonia every year, accounting for almost 1 out of 5 deaths. Pneumonia is usually caused by an air-borne bacterial pathogen.

Symptoms include: fever, cough, and rapid or difficult breathing

Early diagnosis and treatment of pneumonia with simple antibiotics can prevent a large number of deaths. The antibiotics needed to treat 20 children with pneumonia costs only $5.

The three main ways to prevent pneumonia from developing are the following:
- Adequate nutrition, including breastfeeding infants and zinc intake.
- Raising immunization rates.
- Reducing indoor air pollution.

Diarrhea: Millions of people do not have access to safe water and adequate sanitation, which increases their risk of contracting food- and water-borne diarrheal infections. Children are more vulnerable than adults to the effects of diarrhea, because their immune systems are less able to respond to infections that cause diarrhea. Severe diarrhea in children may quickly lead to death.

Nearly all deaths from diarrhea can be prevented through the use of an inexpensive solution of glucose and sodium, which rehydrates the body.

To prevent exposure to the pathogens responsible for diarrhea, developing countries need to focus on the following:

- Sanitation
- Hygiene, especially hand washing
- Access to clean water
- Access to safe food
- Improved nutritional status

Measles is caused by a virus and is easily spread from person to person by contact with nasal or throat secretions through sneezing or coughing of infected persons. Until recently, measles killed nearly 900,000 children throughout the world every year. Following a joint WHO and UNICEF plan to expand the provision of measles vaccines, deaths from measles have declined.

Symptoms include: a high fever, coughing, a runny nose, and a generalized rash
Complications that can develop: pneumonia, diarrhea, malnutrition, and death
Prevention includes: vaccination, which is unavailable in many underdeveloped countries

Malaria: Four parasites cause malaria, and all are transmitted through the bite of an *Anopheles* mosquito. The majority of deaths from malaria occur among young children.

Symptoms include: fever, headache, and vomiting
Prevention includes: the use of insecticide-treated bed nets and indoor spraying with insecticides to prevent mosquito bites
(Yet only 1 out of 25 children in sub-Saharan Africa sleeps under an insecticide-treated bed net.)

Solutions to Decreasing Deaths Globally of Children:

- Just 4 cents can protect and boost one child's immune system with vitamin A capsules.
- Just 6 cents can buy one packet of oral rehydration salts for one child for the treatment of severe dehydration and diarrhea, a leading cause of death among young children.
- Just $1 can buy 40 liters of safe drinking water, which is enough for one child to survive for 40 days, or for 40 children to have safe drinking water for one day.
- Just $5 can provide a box of 100 disposable syringes for use during immunization campaigns, and $17 can immunize one child for life against six deadly diseases.

- Just $100 can provide 10 families with insecticide-treated bed nets to protect them from malaria-carrying mosquitoes.

Major Causes of Child Deaths and the Cost to Treat or Prevent Illness

Disease	Percentage of deaths under five	Number of deaths annually	Cost to treat/prevent illness for one child
Pneumonia	19%	2 million	Antibiotic treatment $0.30
Diarrhea	17%	1.8 million	Oral rehydration packet $0.20
Malaria	8%	850,000	Insecticide treated bed net $5.00
Measles	4%	400,000	Measles vaccine $1.10
HIV/AIDS	3%	350,000	Anti-retroviral drug $5.00

Source: Global Health Council www.globalhealth.org

Cholera in Haiti

Since 2010, an outbreak of cholera has been ongoing in Haiti. **Cholera** is a bacterial disease that causes diarrhea and dehydration. It is spread through the ingestion of contaminated food or drinking water by the feces of an infected person or by untreated sewage. Food is often contaminated by water containing cholera bacteria or by being handled by a person ill with cholera.

Women in Crisis Globally

Did You Know?

- Of the 1.3 billion people living in poverty around the world, about 70% are women.
- Women do about 66% of the work throughout the world in exchange for less than 5% of its income.
- In the least-developed countries, nearly twice as many women as men over age 15 are illiterate.
- Two-thirds of children who do not have access to primary education are girls, and 75% of the world's 876 million illiterate adults are women.
- More than half a million women die during pregnancy and childbirth every year, which equals one death every minute. Of these deaths, 99% occur in developing countries. In parts of Africa, the maternal mortality rate is about 1 out of 16 women.
- Only 28 out of 100 women giving birth are attended by trained health personnel in the least-developed countries.

Major Causes of Death for Women in the United States

1. Heart disease
2. Cancer
3. Stroke
4. Chronic lower-respiratory diseases
5. Alzheimer's disease
6. Unintentional injuries
7. Diabetes
8. Influenza and pneumonia
9. Kidney disease
10. Septicemia

In the United States, the biggest threats to women's health are largely preventable.

1. *To prevent heart disease:*
   - Don't smoke. Avoid exposure to secondhand smoke.
   - Eat a healthful diet that is rich in vegetables, fruits, whole grains, fiber, and fish. Reduce your intake of foods high in saturated fats and sodium.
   - If you have high cholesterol or high blood pressure, carefully follow your doctor's treatment recommendations.
   - Include physical activity in your daily routine.
   - Maintain a healthful weight.
   - If you drink alcohol, do so only in moderation. Too much alcohol can raise blood pressure.
   - If you have diabetes, keep your blood sugar under control.
   - Manage stress.

2. *To reduce the risk of cancer:*
   - Don't smoke. Avoid exposure to secondhand smoke.
   - Include physical activity in your daily routine.
   - Maintain a healthful weight.
   - Eat a healthful diet that is rich in fruits and vegetables, and avoid high-fat foods.
   - Limit your exposure to the sun. When you are outdoors, use sunscreen.
   - If you drink alcohol, do so only in moderation.
   - Consult your doctor for regular cancer screenings.
   - Reduce exposure to cancer-causing substances (carcinogens), such as radon, asbestos, radiation, and air pollution.

3. *To reduce your risk of stroke:*
   - Don't smoke.
   - Limit the amount of saturated fats and cholesterol in your diet. Avoid trans fat entirely.

- Maintain a healthful weight.
- Include physical activity in your daily routine.
- If you have diabetes, keep your blood sugar under control.
- If you drink alcohol, do so only in moderation.

Causes of Death for Women Globally in Low Income Countries
1. HIV/AIDS
2. Maternal conditions
3. Unintentional injuries

Levels of maternal mortality reflect the disparities between the rich and the poor. Inadequate access to prenatal care, poverty, and gender inequality are the main causes of maternal mortality.

Factors for maternal mortality include the following:
- Inadequate access to reproductive health services
- Unsafe abortions (43 million women have abortions; of these, half are unsafe)
- Inadequate prenatal care
- Forced sex and inability to negotiate condom use
- Gender inequalities

Pregnancy and Childbirth

Complications from pregnancy are the leading cause of death for young women ages 15 through 19 in low- and middle-income countries. Throughout the world, 200 million women wish to avoid or delay pregnancy, but they do not have access to modern methods of contraception.

Maternal health and the health of the child are closely related. A child whose mother dies has a risk of death that is three to ten times greater than the risk for a child whose mother is alive. Every year, more than 50 million women, including 60 percent of women in sub-Saharan Africa and 70 percent in South Asia, give birth at home without the help of a trained attendant, which endangers the health of both the mothers and their newborns.

The most common cause of maternal death is bleeding, which can cause death even for a healthy woman within two hours if it is not attended to. Timely and competent care is the key to saving the life of a woman who is hemorrhaging after giving birth. Sepsis and unsafe abortions are the second and third most frequent causes of maternal deaths worldwide.

Access to Birth Control

An estimated 150 million women worldwide do not have access to the birth control that they desire. As a result, many women or girls have babies at young ages they cannot care for, or they have illegal abortions that often are fatal for the women.

Factors for barriers to birth control:
- Lack of education about contraception
- Limited choices
- High costs
- Limited supplies

- Distance to services
- Cultural, religious, or personal objections

In many cultures and regions of the world, the right of a woman to choose when and how many children she will have is viewed as someone else's decision or right.

Women and Anemia

Anemia is a deficiency of red blood cells and/or hemoglobin that decreases the ability of the blood to transfer oxygen to the tissues in the body. Anemia is most prevalent among women, infants, and children because pregnancy and growth increase the body's demand for iron. The WHO estimates that 2 billion people in the world are anemic.

Approximately half of all cases of anemia are a result of dietary iron deficiency caused by an inadequate intake of and poor absorption of iron. Anemia also can be caused by infections, malaria, genetic disorders such as sickle cells, and blood loss during childbirth.

Interventions to decrease anemia among women include the following:

- Iron supplements for pregnant women and adolescent girls
- The reduction of malaria and hookworms
- Efforts to ensure that a mother leaves adequate time between the births of children, as a mother who gives birth too soon after a previous birth can suffer severe anemia and can bleed to death.

Gender-Based Violence

A major public health and human rights concern in many societies throughout the world is **gender-based violence**. Rape, domestic violence, child marriage, sex trafficking, and female genital mutilation are just a few of the abuses that women and girls are forced to suffer. Wars are currently raging in many parts of the world, and about 90 percent of those injured or killed in these conflicts are civilians, 75 percent of whom are women and children. Millions of women caught up in the midst of wars are raped or forced to endure other types of violence, displaced from their own homes, lose loved ones, or are suddenly forced to become the sole provider for their families.

Violence against women is one of the four general causes of death in the world today, along with disease, hunger, and war, according to the head of a Swiss defense institute that recently published a study entitled, "Women in an Insecure World." Swiss Ambassador Theodor Winkler, Director of the Geneva Center for the Democratic Control of Armed Forces, has stated that the number of women who die as a result of gender-related violence, deprivation, and discrimination is greater than the number of casualties in all the wars of the twentieth century combined.

Winkler went on to say that approximately 80 million of the 200 million missing females are the result of abortions of female fetuses in societies in which boys have a higher value than girls. The report notes that medical testing for **sex selection**, although it has been officially banned, has become "a booming business" in China, India, and South Korea, all of which now have significantly fewer girls than boys.

The World Health Organization's World Report on Violence and Health notes that one of the most common forms of violence against women is domestic violence. This type of violence is frequently invisible because it happens behind closed doors in the privacy of homes, and many legal systems and cultural norms do not treat such violence as crimes, but rather as "private" family matters or a normal part of domestic life.

An **honor killing** is a murder of a woman who has been perceived as having brought dishonor to her family. Honor killings are typically committed by the victim's own relatives and/or community, and, unlike crimes of passion or rage-induced killings, they are usually planned in advance. An **honor suicide** occurs when a woman who is considered to be disgraced is ordered or pressured into killing herself. Hundreds, if not thousands, of women are murdered by their families every year for the sake of family "honor." This practice cuts across some cultures and religions. Honor killings occur in Bangladesh, Brazil, Ecuador, Egypt, India, Israel, Jordan, Pakistan, Morocco, Turkey, Uganda, Iran, and Iraq. It is estimated that every day in Pakistan, at least three women are victims of honor killings, and in India, more than 5,000 brides die annually because their dowries are considered to be insufficient.

Honor killings are performed for a wide variety of reasons. Marital infidelity, pre-marital sex, flirting, and even failing to serve a meal on time can all be perceived as bringing shame upon a family. Amnesty International even reported one case in which a husband murdered his wife based on a dream that she had betrayed him. In Turkey, a young woman's throat was cut in a public square because a love ballad had been dedicated to her on the radio.

Female Genital Mutilation

Female genital mutilation, often referred to as female circumcision, involves the partial or complete removal of the external female genitalia or other injuries to female genital organs for cultural, religious, or other non-medical reasons. Today, the number of girls and women who have undergone female genital mutilation is between 100 and 140 million. It is estimated that a further 2 million girls are currently at risk of having to undergo this mutilating procedure.

Most girls and women who have undergone genital mutilation live in 28 African countries, although some live in Asia and the Middle East. In addition, some immigrants from these countries and regions to Europe, Australia, Canada, and the United States also have undergone this procedure, which is usually performed by a traditional practitioner with instruments such as knives and other blades and without any type of anesthetic. The age at which female genital mutilation is performed varies from infants who are only a few days old, to female children and adolescents and, occasionally, to mature women. Refusal to undergo the procedure may jeopardize a woman's family relationships, her social life, and her ability to find a spouse.

Female genital mutilation is performed for the following reasons:

- To maintain chastity and virginity before marriage and fidelity during marriage
- To increase male sexual pleasure
- To have females identify with their cultural heritage
- External female genitalia are considered dirty and unsightly
- The notion that women's bodies are inherently flawed and require correction.

Health Consequences of Female Genital Mutilation:

- Severe pain
- Shock
- Hemorrhage
- Ulceration of the genital region and injury to adjacent tissue
- Infection that can cause death
- Cysts and abscesses

- Scar formation
- Damage to the urethra, resulting in urinary incontinence
- Pain during sexual intercourse and sexual dysfunction
- Difficulties with childbirt
- Possible transmission of HIV when one instrument is used in multiple operations.

Genital mutilation can leave lasting marks on the lives and minds of women who have undergone it. In the long term, these women may suffer feelings of incompleteness, anxiety, and depression.

Ending Female Genital Mutilation

The Torture Convention defines **torture** as "any act by which severe pain or suffering, whether physical or mental, is intentionally inflicted on a person." An unauthorized invasion or alteration of a person's body represents a disregard for that person's fundamental right. Respect for women's dignity implies acceptance of their physical qualities, including the natural appearance of their genitalia and their normal sexual functions. A decision to alter those qualities should not be imposed upon a woman or girl for the purpose of reinforcing socially defined roles. Similarly, because female genital mutilation is an invasion into one of the most intimate aspects of a woman's life, her sexuality, the practice of genital mutilation violates her rights to privacy. It is also a form of violence against women, because in some cases it is performed despite a woman's protests or before she has attained the age of consent, which varies among different countries.

Violence against women is being addressed at the international level as a human rights issue. UNICEF and the United Nations Development Fund for Women have programs in place that address the issue. However, much work needs to be done at local levels. Increased public awareness and greater education about female genital mutilation is definitely needed.

Human Trafficking

Human trafficking for the purpose of sexual exploitation has become a part of international organized crime and generates high profits with low risks for traffickers. The United Nations estimates that 4 million people are bought and sold each year, resulting in $7 billion in profits to criminal organizations. Many countries have no laws or very weak ones against human trafficking, thus making it less risky and more profitable to criminals than trafficking in drugs or weapons. Trafficking networks may buy, abduct, or lure girls and women with promises of a better life in another country, only to transport them to places where they essentially work as slaves in forced prostitution, sweatshop labor, and in private homes as servants.

Several factors lead women to look for potential work in other countries. Globalization has resulted in an increase in poverty among females, forcing greater numbers of women in various countries to emigrate in search of work. Seeking job opportunities abroad, some women turn to newspaper ads, acquaintances, marriage agencies, labor recruiters, and modeling agencies; which many times intentionally mislead these women and trick them into accepting positions as nannies, maids, dancers, factory workers, and hostesses. These positions often are fake; the women are transported to another country, where they do not speak the language, their passports have been taken, and they end up as slaves.

Trafficking in women has been increasing in Eastern Europe, particularly Ukraine, and in Africa and Southeast Asia, from which countries the women are transported to North America. The majority of child trafficking occurs in Asia, although it is a global problem. In Thailand, up to one-third of prostitutes are children and adolescents under the age of 18. Nepal's extreme poverty and its economic and political relationship with India have facilitated the trafficking of Nepali women and girls to brothels in India.

Debt bondage is a situation in which debtors pledge their personal services against a debt that they owe, but the person to whom they owe the debt fails to deduct the value of their services from the debt, or does not limit and define the length and nature of those services. For example, if a mother with no money has a child who is ill and in need of medicine, she might get a loan from one of those debtors and will then be forced to pay off the debt by becoming a slave. Unfortunately, the debtors ensure that the debts are never paid off.

Ending Human Trafficking

Federal trafficking legislation has only been in place in the United States since 2000. It provides for strict penalties for human traffickers and gives victims a variety of benefits, including a special temporary visa for three years. A victim can receive medical counseling, psychological counseling, and emergency shelter. However, to receive these benefits, a victim must testify against her traffickers—something that most girls and women, out of fear of retaliation, will not do. Although the 2000 laws are a start, more pressure must be placed on the federal government to protect and aid the victims of human trafficking without penalties.

Ending Gender-based Violence

Much violence is tied into the economic slavery of women. Millions of women in the world are plagued by not having enough money to live on, which keeps them imprisoned in violent relationships. Jobs that provide living wages need to be created for women to help them become independent. Another means of help is to assist women with planning their families and futures. Family planning services allow women to decide if, when, and how often they wish to have children.

Family planning funding has decreased by about 40 percent in real terms since 1995. At the same time, the adolescent population has grown and is expected to continue to do so over the next two decades. Family planning programs reduce maternal and newborn mortality, unintended pregnancies, and incidences of unsafe abortions.

> The problems we face today, violent conflicts, destruction of nature, poverty, hunger and so on, are human-created problems which can be resolved through human effort, understanding and the development of a sense of brotherhood and sisterhood. We need to cultivate a universal responsibility for one another and the planet we share.
>
> —*the Dalai Lama*

Decreasing the devastating impact of infectious diseases can prevent deaths and improve the quality of lives throughout the world. Proven and cost-effective medicines, vaccines, and other products and methods do exist to prevent and treat illnesses.

Some of the best health care solutions are as simple and inexpensive as teaching mothers to keep their newborns clean and warm, advising people at risk of heart disease to eat a low-fat diet, and educating people about the importance of using condoms to avoid being infected with HIV. Many health care interventions—such as curbing tobacco use and improving nutrition—target several health problems at once.

The most cost-effective interventions include the following:

- **Provide bed nets** treated with insecticide ($4.80 per bed net). Malaria is transmitted by mosquitoes almost exclusively at night. Bed nets have been proven to control the spread of the disease in endemic regions.

- **Provide water purification systems** ($0.04 per sachet). More than one billion people in the world do not have access to safe drinking water. Simple household water treatments can stop the spread of deadly water-borne diseases such as cholera. PUR packets from Procter and Gamble are very effective in purifying drinking water in developing countries.

- **Increase condom availability** ($1 or less per condom). Prevention is still the best way to stop the spread of HIV and STDs. Behavioral changes and condom use can decrease the global pandemic of HIV/AIDS.

- **Vaccinate poor children against measles** ($0.13 per dose). The measles vaccine is safe, inexpensive, and almost 100% effective. Yet in many developing countries, children still do not have access to these vaccines, and, as a result, 500,000 to 700,000 children die each year from this preventable disease, while many others suffer lifelong disabilities, including blindness, deafness, and brain damage.

- **Tax tobacco products** to increase their price and thus motivate people to quit smoking, which will reduce the prevalence of cardiovascular disease, cancer, and respiratory diseases. Tobacco is the second major cause of death in the world—killing one in 10 adults worldwide, or about 5 million people each year.

- **Attack the spread of HIV** by promoting condom use among populations at high risk; treating other sexually-transmitted diseases; providing antiretroviral medications, especially for pregnant women; and offering voluntary HIV/AIDS counseling and testing.

- **Make sure that children and pregnant women receive essential nutrients**, including vitamin A, iron, and iodine to prevent maternal anemia, infant deaths, and other long-term health problems.

- **Treat TB patients** with antibiotics and short-term chemotherapy.

- **Promote the use of aspirin** in adults and behavioral changes such as a healthful diet and exercise to treat and prevent heart attacks and strokes.

References:

Abreu, A. G., Noguer, I., and Cowgill, K. "HIV/AIDS in Latin American Countries," The World Bank, http://go.worldbank.org/KIC4QIMK20

A Joint Assessment of HIV/AIDS Prevention, Treatment and Care in China. State Council HIV/AIDS Working Committee Office and UN Theme Group on HIV/AIDS in China, 2003. http://www.unaids.org.cn/uploadfiles/20080725151739.pdf

Bryce, J., Boschi-Pinto, C., Shibuya, K., and Black, R. E. WHO Child Health Epidemiology Reference Group: "WHO estimates the causes of death in children," *Lancet*, 365(9465) (2005): 1147-1152.

BBC News, "Cuba to help Caribbean fight AIDS," July 16, 2004.

Bogart, L. M. and Thorburn, S. "Are HIV/AIDS conspiracy beliefs a barrier to HIV prevention among African Americans?" *Journal of Acquired Immune Deficiency Syndromes*, 38(2) (2005): 213-218.

Bronfman, M. N., et al. "Mobile populations and HIV/AIDS in Central America and Mexico: research for action," *AIDS*: vol. 16 Supplement 3, December 2002, S42-S49.

Campbell, O. M. R. and Graham, W. J. "Strategies for reducing maternal mortality: getting on with what works," *Lancet*, 368 (2006): 2121-2122.

Centers for Disease Control and Prevention. *HIV/AIDS Surveillance Report* 7 (2). Atlanta: U.S. Department of Health and Human Services, Centers for Disease Control and Prevention, 1995, http://www.cdc.gov/hiv/stats/hasrlink.htm.

Centers for Disease Control and Prevention. *HIV/AIDS Among African Americans Fact Sheet*, Atlanta: U.S. Department of Health and Human Services, Centers for Disease Control and Prevention, 2005, http:/Jwww.cdc.gov/hiv/.

Centers for Disease Control and Prevention. *HIV/AIDS Surveillance Report 15*, Atlanta: U.S. Department of Health and Human Services, Centers for Disease Control and Prevention, 2003, http://www.cdc.gov/hiv/stats/.

Centers for Disease Control and Prevention. *HIV/AIDS among Youth Fact Sheet*, Atlanta: U.S. Department of Health and Human Services, Centers for Disease Control and Prevention, 2005, http://www.cdc.gov/hiv/pubs/facts/youth.htm.

CDC. "Monitoring selected national HIV prevention and care objectives by using HIV surveillance data—United States and 6 U.S. dependent areas—2010." *HIV Surveillance Supplemental Report 2012*, 17(No. 3, part A), Published June 2012. http://www.cdc.gov/hiv/pdf/statistics_2010_HIV_Surveillance_Report_vol_17_no_3.pdf.

CDC. "Estimated HIV incidence in the United States, 2007–2010." *HIV Surveillance Supplemental Report 2012*, 17(No. 4). Published December 2012. http://www.cdc.gov/hiv/surveillance/resources/reports/2010supp_vol17no4/.

CDC. *HIV Surveillance Report, 2010*; vol. 22. Published March 2012. http://www.cdc.gov/hiv/library/reports/surveillance/2011/surveillance_Report_vol_23.html.

Centers for Disease Control and Prevention. *HIV/AIDS Among Women Fact Sheet*, Atlanta: U.S. Department of Health and Human Services, Centers for Disease Control and Prevention, 2004, http://www.cdc .gov/hiv/pubs/facts/women.htm.

Centers for Disease Control and Prevention. *HIV/AIDS Among Men Who Have Sex with Men Fact Sheet*, Atlanta: U.S. Department of Health and Human Services, Centers for Disease Control and Prevention, 2005.

Centers for Disease Control and Prevention, *HIV/AIDS Surveillance Report, 2005*, vol. 17, Atlanta: U.S. Department of Health and Human Services, CDC, 2006, 1-46.

Channel 4, UK, *Dying for Drugs*, April 27, 2003.

Cohen, J. "The overlooked epidemic," *Science*, vol. 313 Issue 5786, July 28, 2006.

Cohen, J. "Mexico: Prevention programs target migrants," *Science*, vol. 313 Issue 5786, July 28, 2006.

Cohen, J. "Haiti: Making headway under hellacious circumstances," *Science*, vol. 313 Issue 5786, July 28, 2006.

Colgan, Ann-Louise. "Hazardous to health: The World Bank and IMF in Africa," *Africa Action*, April 18, 2002.

DeParle, J. "Talk of government being out to get blacks falls on more attentive ears," *The New York Times*, Oct. 29, 1990.

Disease Control Priorities Project. "Best buys and priorities for action in developing countries," *Investing in Global Health*, April 2006.

Fawthrop, T, "Cuba: Is it a model in HIV/AIDS battle?" *London Panos*, 2003, at http://panos.org.uk/features/cuba-is-it-a-model-in-the-hivaids-battle/

Fink, S. "Cuba's energetic AIDS doctor," *American Journal of Public Health*, 93(5) (2003): 712-716.

Frasca, T. (2005). *AIDS in Latin America*, Basingstoke, England: Palgrave/Macmillan, 144.

Goldstein, M. A. "The biological roots of heat-of-passion crimes and honor killings," *Politics and the Life Sciences*, vol. 21, no 2, September 2002, 28-37.

Ghosh, T. K. "AIDS: A serious challenge to public health," *Journal of the Indian Medical Association*, 84(1) (1986): 29-30.

Hacker, M., Malta, M., Enriquez, M., et al. "Human immunodeficiency virus, AIDS, and drug consumption in South America and the Caribbean: Epidemiological evidence and initiatives to curb the epidemic," *Rev Panam Salud Publica*, 18(4/5) (2005): 303-313.

Henry J. Kaiser Foundation. *Global Health Facts*, 2009. http://www.KaiserEDU.org

Human Rights Watch. "Jordan Parliament Supports Impunity for Honor Killing," Press Release, Washington, D.C.: January 2000.

Jamison, D. T., Breman, J. G., Measham, A. R., Alleyne, G., Claeson, M., Evans, D. B., Jha, P., Mills, A., and Musgrove, P. *Disease Control Priorities in Developing Countries* (2nd ed.), New York: Oxford University Press, 2006.

Jamison, D.T., et al. *Priorities in Health*, Washington, D.C.: World Bank, 2006.

Jarosewich, I. "Reports on trafficking of women in Europe: Most who seek rescue are from Ukraine," *The Ukrainian Weekly*, no. 32, vol. LXVI, August 9, 1998, at http://www.ukrweekly.com/Archive/1998/329802.shtnil.

Kanics, J. "Trafficking in Women," *Global Survival Network*, eds. Tom Barry (LRC) and Martha Honey (IPS) *In Focus*, 3(30) (October 1998), at http://www.foreignpolicyinfocus.or Jbriefs/vol3/v3n30wom.html.

Kanics, J. "Foreign Policy in Focus: Trafficking in Women," *Global Survival Network*, vol. 3, no. 30, October 1998.

Kakar, D. N. and Kakar, S. N. *Combating AIDS in the 21st century: Issues and challenges*, New Delhi: Sterling Publishers LLC, 31, 2001.

Lawn, J. E., Cousens, S, Darmstadt, G. L., Bhutta, Z., Martines, J., Paul, V, et al. "1 year after The Lancet Neonatal Survival Series—was the call for action heard?" *Lancet*, 367 (2006): 1541-1547.

Lawn, J. E., Cousens, S., and Zupan, J. "4 million neonatal deaths: When? where? why?" *Lancet*, 365 (2005): 891-900.

Lopez, A. D., Mathers, C. D., Ezzati, M., Jamison, D. T., and Murray, C. J. L. *Global Burden of Disease and Risk Factors*, New York: Oxford University Press, 2006.

National Alliance of State and Territorial AIDS Directors. *HIV/AIDS: African American Perspectives and Recommendations for State and Local AIDS Directors and Health Departments*, 2001.

Bilefsky, D. "How to avoid honor killing in Turkey? Honor Suicide," *New York Times*, at http://www.nytimes.com/2006/07/16/world/europe/16turkey.html?pagewanted=all. (July 16, 2006).

Pope, Victoria. "Trafficking in women: Procuring Russians for sex abroad—even in America." *US News and World Report*, April 7, 1997, at htp://www.usnews.cornIusnews/issue/970407/7ring.htm.

Ronsmans, C. and Graham, W. J. "Maternal mortality: Who, when, where and why." *The Lancet*, 368 (2006): 1189-1199.

Black, R. E., Morris, S. S., and Bryce, J. "Where and why are 10 million children dying every year?" *The Lancet*, vol. 361, no. 9376, June 28, 2003.

Specter, M. "Contraband women—A special report: Traffickers' new cargo: Naive slavic women," *The New York Times*, January 11, 1998.

The Hemy J. Kaiser Family Foundation and the National Alliance of State and Territorial AIDS Directors. *National ADAP Monitoring Project*, Annual Report, 2005, at http://www.kff.org/hivaids/7288.cfm.

The Kaiser Family Foundation. *Kaiser Family Foundation Survey of Americans on HIV/A1DS: Part Three—Experiences and Opinions by Race/Ethnicity and Age*, August 2004, at http://www.kff.org/hivaids/upload/44743_l.pdf.

The Kaiser Family Foundation. *African Americans and HIV/AIDS*, HIV/AIDS Policy Fact Sheet, Feb. 2005, at http://www.kff.org/hivaidsl.

The Kaiser Family Foundation. *The Uninsured: A Primer - Key Facts About Americans Without Health Insurance*, Nov. 2004, at http://www.kff.org/uninsured/72l6.cfm?\.

"Spreading the word about HIV/AIDS in India," *The Lancet*, vol. 361, May 3, 2003.

The Rutherford Institute 4/10/06 at http:/Jwww.rutherford.orglarticles_db/commentary.asp?record_id=397

UNAIDS/WHO 2006 AIDS epidemic update at http://www.unaids.org/en/KnowledgeCentre/HIVData/EpiUpdate/EpiUpdArchive/2006/default.asp

UNAIDS, *A Study of the Pan Caribbean Partnership against HIV/AIDS (PANCAP) Common Goals, Shared Responses*, December, 2004, at http://data.unaids.org/publications/IRC-pub06/jc1089-pancap_en.pdf

UNAIDS, *UNAIDS at Country Level: Progress Report 2004* at http://data.unaids.org/pub/Report/2006/2006_country_progress_report_burundi_en.pdf

UNICEF, *State of the World's Children*, 2005-2007, at http://www.unicef.org/eapro/Human_Development_in_Crisis.pdf

UNICEF, "Statistics: Under 5 Mortality Rate," at http://www.childinfo.org/areas/childmortality/u5data.php.

UNESCO, *EFA Global Monitoring Report*, Paris: UNESCO, 2007.

U.S. Department of Justice, *Bureau of Justice Statistics Bulletin: Prison and Jail Inmates at Midyear 2004*, Washington, D.C.: U.S. Department of Justice, 2005, at http://www.ojp.usdoj.gov/bjs/.

U.S. Department of Health and Human Services, "China urges needle exchanges, free condoms in new AIDS strategy," Associated Press, 7 June 2005.

U.S. Department of Justice (2004, December), *Bureau of Justice Statistics Bulletin: HIV in Prisons and Jails, 2002*, at http://www.ojp.usdoj .gov/bjs/pub/pdf7hivpj02 .pdf

Wongsrichanalai, C., Barcus, M. J., Muth, S., Sutamihardja, A., and Wernsdorfer, W. H. (2007). "A review of malaria diagnostic tools: microscopy and rapid diagnostic test (RDT)." *Am J Trop Med Hyg*, 77 (Suppl 6): 119-27.

World Bank (2000). "Thailand's Response to AIDS: Building on Success, Confronting the Future," *Thailand social Monitor V*, p.10-11 .

World Development Index 2002, The World Bank.

World Health Organization, *Fact sheet N° 104*, March 2007, at http://www.who.org

World Health Organization, "Economic costs of malaria," November 27, 2005.

World Health Organization, "Towards Universal Access: Scaling up priority HIV/AIDS interventions in the health sector," 17 April 2007.

WHO, 2005. *Make every mother and child count*. Geneva: WHO.

WHO, 2005. *Facts and figures form the World Health Report 2005*. Geneva: WHO.

Women's Human Rights Resources at http://www.law-lib.utoronto.caiDianai

Zipperer, M. (July 2005), "HIV/AIDS Prevention and Control: the Cuban Response," *The Lancet Infectious Diseases*, Volume 5, Issue 7.

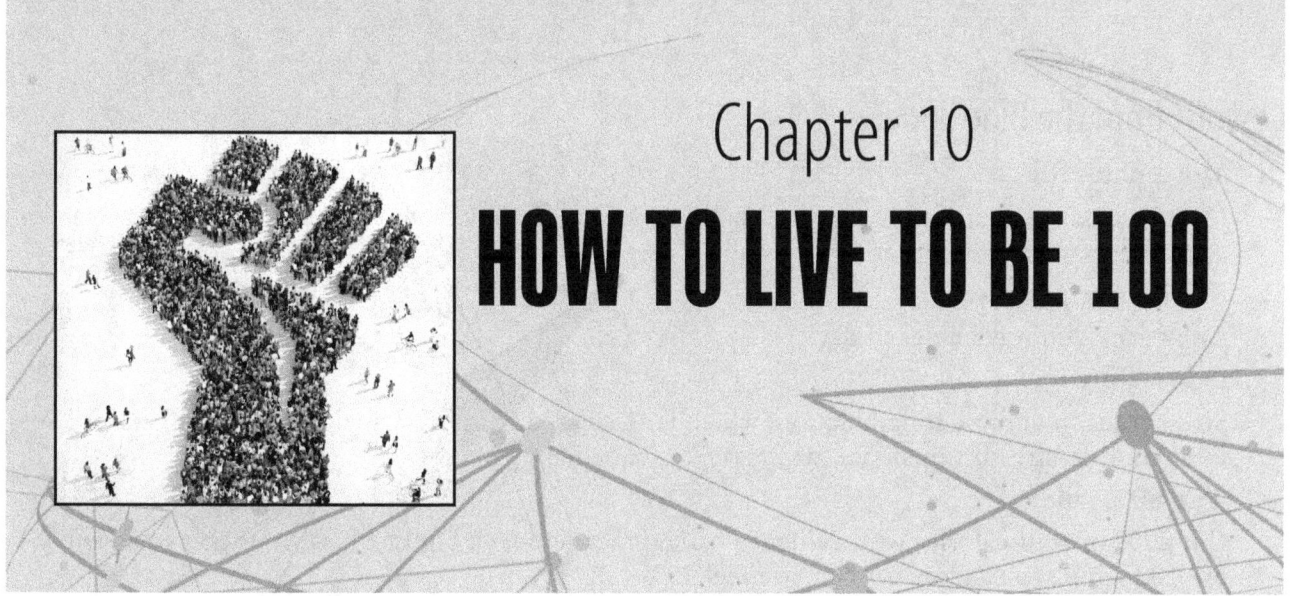

Chapter 10

HOW TO LIVE TO BE 100

Blue Zones are places around the world where people are recorded to live longer. There are less middle-aged onset of preventable diseases like heart disease and adult onset (type 2) diabetes, and premature death. There are many people recorded in these areas that live into their 100's (centurions).

These places are:

1. Sardinia, Italy
2. Okanawa, Japan
3. Loma Linda, California, United States
4. Ikaria, Greece
5. Nicoya, Coast Rica

Ninety percent of longevity has to do with lifestyle, the other 10 percent or less is genetics.

- All Blue Zone areas consume a cup of beans of some type per day. They also consume at least ¼ cup of greens each day and some type of fermented foods like tofu, 90 to 100 percent of Blue Zone Diets are plant based, 65 percent of their diets are high in starches (so much for the low carb. diet idea). Sweet potatoes are a staple in some Blue Zones. All areas consume high amounts of whole grains. Blue Zone meals are large in the morning, medium for lunch, and light for dinner. The old adage of: Eat like a King at breakfast, a Prince at lunch, and a Pauper at dinner holds true. Blue Zone citizens walk often and don't sit for more than 20 minutes or so at a time. Their lives are structured in a way that they are constantly moving. They don't have modern technologies or other conveniences in their lives. Longevity is not sought after in the Blue Zones. They don't go to the gym and rigorously exercise! They also don't take a bunch of supplements, they get all of their nutrition from their foods.

- No cow's milk or cheese is consumed AT ALL in Blue Zones.

- Isolation is harmful to longevity. Having a community that you belong to of some type creates a "sense of belonging." Most Blue Zone citizens and all centurions have a group of friends they have had for most of their lives. Buettner suggests that one should have at least 3 friends that you can count on when you are having a really bad day. Almost all centurions in the Blue Zones had some type of faith-based community that they were part of and participated in faith-based activities or services 4 times monthly. In addition to their friends and faith-based communities, they lived near to their families and the elderly are seen as a vital part of the family unit and participate in daily family activities.

Lessons from the Blue Zone:

1. **Move naturally**

   De-convenience your home, take the stairs, park farther away from the entrance and grow gardens. Have an errand not far away…walk!

2. **Know your purpose**

   Know why you wake up each day!

3. **Down shift**

   Stress leads to chronic inflammation, which is associated with every major age-related disease. Find your de-stressor: meditate, nap, pray, or enjoy happy hour.

4. **The 80% rule**

   Cut 20% of your calories with evidence based practices: eat a big breakfast, eat with your family, use 10 inch plates, and stop when you feel 80% full.

5. **Plant slant**

   Eat a plant-based diet that's heavy on the beans, nuts, and green plants.

6. **Wine at 5**

   Moderate drinkers outlive non-drinkers.

7. **Family first**

   Living in a loving and thriving family can add six years to your ticker! Invest time in your kids, nurture a monogamous relationship, and keep aging parents near by.

8. **Belong**

   It doesn't matter if you're Christian, Buddhist, Muslim, Jewish, or some other religion that meets as a community. Research shows that attending faith-based services four times per month will add 4-14 years of life expectancy.

9. **Right tribe**

   Take stock in who your friends are and extend your social circle to include healthy-minded, supportive people.

Source: https://www.arespectfullife.com/2017/08/19/live-100-blue-zone-way-centurions/

Taking Health Back into Your Own Hands

Each person is ultimately in charge of his or her own health care, and everyone wants the best medical care possible. A proactive patient is an informed patient, one who finds a good doctor and medical facilities, does independent research using reliable sources, and asks detailed, relevant questions of health care experts. The relationship between a patient and his or her doctors should be a partnership in which communication in central.

A proactive patient has three main attributes:

- Knowledge about one's own health problems
- Assertiveness
- Willingness to participate in informed decision-making about one's own health care

Providers must be sensitive to patients' beliefs and cultural values as they collaborate about health decisions. Proactive patients take some responsibility for obtaining their own information about health care so that it is accessible to them, and they understand their own health histories. Proactive patients engage in self-advocacy by being their own advocates: they represent their own interests in the health care decision-making process by asking key questions, searching for information, and ensuring that they receive proper care.

How to get the most from your health care by being a proactive patient:

- Know your rights as a patient.
- Find out about informed-consent procedures, living wills, the durable power of attorney, organ donation, and other legal issues *before* you become ill.
- Ask about alternative procedures and about your treatment plans.

Possible Solutions to Achieve Equality in Health

The quality of health care services that are provided to minority groups and immigrants remains a major challenge in the United States.

Culturally Competent Healthcare

Cultural competence is a set of skills, attitudes, and knowledge that enables people and organizations to work effectively with a diversity of ethnic, racial, and social groups. The existence of racial disparities in the incidences and prevalence of diseases, as well as health status, indicates that a system has not effectively responded to all the groups within a population.

The answers to the following questions can help determine whether or not a health care system in a community is culturally competent.

- Are staff members adequately trained to work with the diverse populations within the community that is being served?
- Can patients make a choice about whether they can see a provider from their own culture?
- Are beneficiaries from minority populations receiving critical and relevant interventions that address disparities?
- Are surveys reaching out to non-English speaking populations and trying to serve them?
- Do community outreach and education programs address disparities that are prevalent within the diverse populations of the community?
- Is there funding to support the institutionalization of cultural competence within the system or organization?
- Does the system or organization welcome and reach out to racial and ethnic groups in the target area?
- Is there diversity and representation of minority professionals and managers within the system or organization?

Solutions to End Health Disparities among Subpopulations

- To reduce many disparities in the health status of different groups of the American population, it is essential to address the issue of poverty.
- Universal health care services would significantly improve the health of those in minority groups and would narrow the gap in the health status between minorities and the general population.
- People and communities must be empowered to pursue solutions to their own problems by acquiring the following:
    - **Social power:** information, skills, and participation in social organizations
    - **Political power:** holding one's government accountable by voting and joining political organizations
    - **Psychological power:** self-esteem, which leads to change.
- The promotion of wellness and healthful lifestyles is essential to the reduction and elimination of the unequal burden of disease mortality and morbidity that ethnic and racial groups currently endure. Because their social environment profoundly affects people's health, it is important to establish accessible exercise programs and to work toward decreasing violence in the neighborhoods of minorities.
- In addition to the social environment, the personal choices that people make, including interactions with family, friends, and members of the community are important factors to consider in attempting to eliminate disparities in the health status of ethnic and racial minority groups.
- Public officials should be held to high standards. When communities become actively involved in the political process in their communities, they can avert crises in political leadership. The following are ways in which people can become involved and empowered:
    - Vote.
    - Write or email concerns and opinions to political representatives.
    - Organize letter-writing campaigns and enlist as many other people as possible.
    - Write letters to the editors of local newspapers.
    - Visit the website RESULTS.org, which contains many useful tools that can be adapted to help target politicians and media outlets.
    - Join existing networks, such as the Global Call to Action Against Poverty at http://www.whiteband.org/, which has national chapters in many countries.

Some questions to consider:

- What levels of poverty, hunger, and homelessness can we as a society tolerate, while claiming to be a compassionate country?
- What is the appropriate minimum wage, and how can people with low-paying jobs supplement their incomes?
- What new policy strategies can we develop to address discrimination based on ethnicity, race, and gender that leads to health disparities?
- How can our government provide all of its citizens with the basic human needs: food, shelter, health care, and wages that they can live on?
- How can our country move forward in providing equal opportunities to its most disadvantaged citizens?

Whether you're engaging in personal interactions or working within a system or agency, cultural competence is a fundamental awareness of the language, thoughts, behaviors, and institutions of ethnic, racial, religious, or social groups. Start by exploring your own views, values, and practices and digging deep to address biases, beliefs, and prejudices. The goal is to recognize that what is "normal" to you may look very different to someone else. Cultural competence in health care delivery includes using that awareness to provide culturally appropriate, respectful, and relevant care and education. Health professionals must learn to ask questions, listen carefully, respond to what is said, speak simply and respectfully, and involve clients in their own treatment plans.

••

The right to health does not mean the right to be healthy, nor does it mean that poor
governments must put in place expensive health services for which they have no resources.
But it does require governments and public authorities to put in place policies and action plans
which will lead to available and accessible health care for all in the shortest possible time.
To ensure that this happens is the challenge facing both the human rights community
and public health professionals.
—*United Nations High Commissioner for Human Rights Mary Robinson*

••

Conclusion

It's tough to be a young person today and to look at the problems of the world without completely losing hope. What I have found in my life to help me get through those times is to participate. Anything that you can do to get involved will help you feel more connected to the world. It is precisely during these trying times that the United States needs its best and brightest young people, from all walks of life, to step forward and commit to public service. Times like these call for people to stand up and get to work. To break barriers and to drive change, roll up your sleeves instead of throwing up your hands. Because of globalization, our world is so small that you cannot ignore inhumane circumstances, or the fact that one out of every eight Americans is living in poverty, with millions more struggling just to get by. You cannot turn away as pandemic diseases torment the people of entire continents. And you can't look aside as citizens are denied their most basic human rights, such as safe food, water, and access to health care.

When it comes to public health, lives are often saved, or dramatically improved, by the things that cost the least. Simple undertakings—such as washing hands, using a seatbelt, quitting smoking, eating more fruits and vegetables and less fat and sugar—have little or no cost to an individual. However, collectively, such actions can make a huge difference in public health.

Use your privileged, educated eyes to see the burdens of those who are less privileged and to help them. In whatever career you find yourself, become an agent of change to work toward ensuring that a fair and equal opportunity is available for *all*!

References:

Abramson, J. *Overdosed America: The Broken Promise of American Medicine*, New York: Harper Collins, 2004.

ABC News/Kaiser Family Foundation/*USA Today, Health Care in America 2006 Survey*, October 17, 2006.

Agency for Healthcare Research and Quality. "Out-of-Pocket Expenditures on Health Care and Insurance Premiums among the Non-Elderly Population 2003," March 2006.

Aoki, Naomi. "Journals pool clout to ensure integrity," *The Boston Globe*, September 10, 2001.

Blendon, R.J., et al. "Understanding the American public's priorities: A 2006 perspective," *Health Affairs Web Exclusive* W508, 17 October 2006.

Borger, C., et al. "Health spending projections through 2015: Changes on the horizon," *Health Affairs Web Exclusive* W61, 22 February 2006.

Boston at Risk, *Six Principles for a New Health Care System: A Blue Print for Action*, Families USA, 2006.

California Health Care Foundation, Health Care Costs, Oakland, CA: California Health Care Foundation, March 2, 2005. http://www.chcf.org/topics/healthinsurance/index.cfm?subtopic=CL498&CFNoCache=TRUE&order=alpha

Catlin, A. C., Cowan, S., Heffler, et al. "National Health Spending in 2005," *Health Affairs* 26(1) (2006): 142-153.

Chernew, M. "Rising Health Care Costs and the Decline in Insurance Coverage," *Economic Research Initiative on the Uninsured*, ERTU Working Paper 8, September 2002.

Committee on the Consequences of Uninsurance. *Health Insurance is a Family Matter*, Washington, D.C.: The National Academies Press, 2002.

Eagan, Andrea Boroff. *The Women's Health Movement and Its Lasting Impact, An Unfinished Revolution, Women and Health Care in America*, Emily Friedman (ed.), New York: United Hospital Fund of New York, 1994.

FamiliesUSA, at www.Farniliesusa.org.

Glenmullen, J. *The Antidepressant Solution*, New York: Free Press, 2006.

Health Care for All, *1995-2000 Annual Report*, at www.hcfa.org.

Hewitt Associates, LLC. *Health Care Expectations: Future State and Direction 2005*. November 17, 2004.

Himmelstein, D., Warren, E., Thorne, D., and Woolhander, S. "Illness and Injury as Contributors to Bankruptcy," *Health Affairs Web Exclusive* W5-63, February 2, 2005.

Langill, Donna, et al. *Medicaid Managed Care: An Advocate's Guide for Protecting Children*, Washington, D.C.: National Association of Children's Advocates and National Health Law Program, 1996, 115.

Marone, J. *The Democratic Wish, Popular Participation and the Limits of American Government*, New York: Basic Books, 1990.

McClellan, R. A., Burt, A. D., and Fleming, K. A. "Long-term safety and effectiveness of iron-chelation therapy with deferiprone for thalassemia major," *New England Journal of Medicine*, vol. 339 no. 7 (1998): 417-423.

McKinsey and Company. "Will Health Benefit Costs Eclipse Profits?" *The McKinsey Quarterly Chart Focus Newsletter*, September 2004.

Meredith, J. and Dunham, C. *Real Clout*, Boston: The Access Project, 1999.

Pear, R. "U.S. health care spending reaches all-time high: 15% of GDP," *The New York Times*, January 9, 2004, 3.

Schultz, Stacey. "True, false, whatever," *U.S. News & World Report*, September 17, 2001.

Seto, N. and Weiskopf, B. K. *Community Benefits, Need for Action, an Opportunity for Healthcare Change. A Workbook for Grassroots Leaders and Community Organizations*, Boston: The Access Project, 1998.

Collins, S. R., Davis, K., Doty, M. M., Kriss, J. L., and Holmgren, A. L. "Gaps in health insurance: An all-American problem," New York, NY: The Commonwealth Fund, April 2006.

Starr, P. *The Social Transformation of American Medicine*, New York: Basic Books, 1982.

The Commonwealth Fund, *Wages, Health Benefits, and Workers' Health*, Issue Brief, October 2004.

The Henry J. Kaiser Family Foundation, *Employee Health Benefits: 2006 Annual Survey*, September 26, 2006.

The Henry J. Kaiser Family Foundation, *The Uninsured: A Primer, Key Facts About Americans without Health Insurance 2004*, November 10, 2004.

The Henry J. Kaiser Family Foundation, *Health Care Worries in Context with Other Worries 2004*, October 4, 2004.

POST-TEST

Name_____ Date_____

1. What is the leading cause of death in the U.S and what contributes to getting this disease?

2. Define community, public, and global health.

3. What are factors that contribute to a community's health?

4. Discuss some achievements in public health in the U.S.

5. Define lifestyle diseases and discuss incidence and prevalence.

6. What is primary, secondary, and tertiary prevention of disease?

7. Explain the 3-legged approach to a successful community health campaign.

8. Discuss factors for a country's mortality rate.

9. Why does the U.S. have a high infant mortality rate and a lower life expectancy than other industrialized countries?

10. Explain factory farming and the health of our food supply.

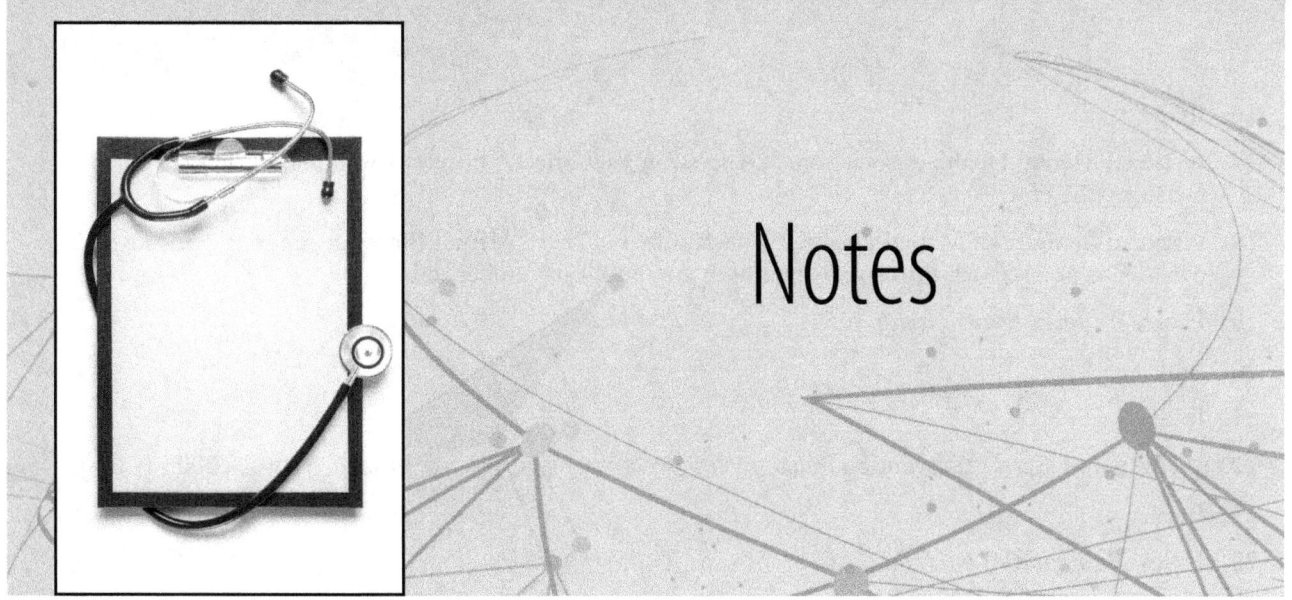

Notes

1. World Health Organization. "Constitution of the World Health Organization." *Chronicle of the World Health Organization*. Geneva, Switzerland: WHO, 1947.

2. U.S. Department of Health and Human Services. *Mental Health: A Report of the Surgeon General: Executive Summary*. Rockville, MD: U.S. Department of Health and Human Services, Substance Abuse and Mental Health Service Administration, Center for Mental Health Services, National Institute of Health, National Institute of Mental Health, 1999.

3. National Center for Statistics and Analysis. "Top 10 Leading Causes of Death in the US for 2002." http://www.nhtsa.dot.gov.

4. Ibid.

5. Healthy People 2020 Fact Sheet. "Healthy People in Healthy Communities." http://www.health.gov.healthypeople.

6. Scanlan, James. "Race and Mortality." *Society*, Vol. 37, No. 2, January 2000.

7. Guyer, Bernard, et al. "Annual Summary of Vital Statistics: Trends in the Health of Americans During the 20th Century." *Pediatrics*, Vol. 106, No. 6, December 2000.

8. Milansky, Aubrey. *Your Genetic Destiny*. New York: Perseus Publishing, 2001.

9. Vitucci, Jeff. "The State of Hispanic Health." *Hispanic Business*, Vol. 21, No. 6, June 1999.

10. World Health Organization. 2004. Why Gender and Health? http://www.who.int/gender/genderandhealth/en.

11. Hales, Dianne. *An Invitation to Health*, 11th ed. Belmont, CA: Thomson/Wadsworth, 2005.

12. National Mental Heath Association. "Mental Health Fact Sheets." http://www.nmha.org/.

13. Ibid.

14. Ibid.

15. Ibid.

16. Ibid.

17. National Mental Health Association. "Depression Fact Sheet." http://www.nmha.org/infoctr/factsheets/21.cfm.

18. National Institute of Mental Health. "The Numbers Count: Mental Illness in America." *Science on Our Minds Fact Sheet Series.* http://www.nimh.nih.gov/publicat/numbers.cfm.

19. Hales, *An Invitation to Health*, p. 57.

20. Ibid.

21. Ibid.

22. Weitzstein, Cheryl. "Preventing Suicide." *Insight in the News*, Vol. 16, No. 16, May 1, 2000.

23. Ibid.

24. Hales, *An Invitation to Health*, p. 62.

25. National Mental Health Association. "Suicide Fact Sheet." http://www.nmha.org/infoctr/factsheets/51.cfm.

26. Ho, Beng-Choon, et al. "Schizophrenia and Other Psychotic Disorders." In *Textbook of Clinical Psychiatry*, 4th ed. Washington, DC: American Psychiatric Publishing, Inc., 2003, p. 379.

27. National Mental Health Association. "Seasonal Affective Disorder Fact Sheet." http://www.nmha.org/infoctr/factsheets/27.cfm.

28. National Institute of Mental Health. "What Is Social Phobia?" http://www.nimh.nih.gov/healthinformation/socialphobiamenu.cfm.

29. Insel, P., and Roth, W., eds. 2006. *Core Concepts in Health*, 10th ed. New York: McGraw-Hill.

30. Dunn, A.L., M.H. Trivedi, J.B. Kampert, C.G. Clark, and H.O. Chambliss. "Exercise Treatment for Depression—Efficacy and Dose Response." *American Journal of Preventive Medicine*. January, 2005.

31. http://www.google.com/search?hl=en&lr=&client=firefox-a&rls=org.mozilla:en-US:official&oi=defmore&defl=en&q=defin:Hormone.

32. http://www.alz.org/Resources/Glossary.asp.

33. Newman, E. *No More Test Anxiety*. Los Angeles, CA: Learning Skills Publications, 1996.

34. http://www.contemplativemind.org/practices/subnav/mindfulness.htm.

35. Ibid.

36. Jacobson, E. *Progressive relaxation*. Chicago: University of Chicago Press, 1938.

37. http://www.ship.edu/~cgboeree/musclerelaxation.html.

38. Booth, Frank, et al. "Physiologists Claim SEDS Is Second Greatest Threat to US Public Health." *Medical Letter on the CDC & FDA*, June 24, 2001.

39. "Physical Activity and Health: Adults," a Report of the Surgeon General, President's Council on Physical Fitness and Sports, http://www.cdc.gov.

40. Grubbs, L., and J. Carter. "The Relationship of Perceived Benefit and Barriers to Reported Exercise Behaviors in College Undergraduates." *Family and Community Health*, Vol. 25, No. 2, July 2002, p. 76.

41. Prochaska, J.O., and C.C. DiClemente. "Transtheoretical Therapy Toward a More Integrative Model of Change." *Psychotherapy: Theory, Research and Practice*, Vol. 19, No. 3, pp. 276–287.

42. Prochaska, J.O., J.C. Norcross, and C.C. DiClemente. *Changing for Good*. New York: William Morrow, 1994.

43. American Heart Association. "A Statement on Exercise: Benefits and Recommendations for Physical Activity Programs for All Americans." *Circulation*, Vol. 91, p. 580.

44. American College of Sports Medicine. *ACSM's Guidelines for Exercise Testing and Prescription*. Baltimore, MD: Lippincott Williams and Wilkins, 2000.

45. American College of Sports Medicine. "Position Stand: The Recommended Quality and Quantity of Exercise for Developing and Maintaining Cardiorespiratory and Muscular Fitness, and Flexibility in Healthy Adults." *Medicine and Science in Sports and Exercise*, Vol. 30, 1998, pp. 975–991.

46. American College of Sports Medicine. http://www.acsm.org.

47. Borg, G. A. "Psychophysical Basis of Perceived Exertion." *Medicine and Science in Sports and Exercise*, Vol. 14, No. 5, 2003, pp. 377–381.

48. Ibid.

49. American College of Sports Medicine. "The Recommended Quantity and Quality of Exercise for Developing and Maintaining Cardiorespiratory and Muscular Fitness and Flexibility in Healthy Adults." *Medicine and Science in Sports and Exercise*, Vol. 30, No. 6, 1998, pp. 975–991.

50. Shrier, I., and K. Gossal. "Myths and Truths of Stretching." *Physician and Sports Medicine*, Vol. 28, No. 8, 2000, pp. 57–63.

51. Thygerson, A. *Fit to Be Well: Essential Concepts*. Sudbury, MA: Jones and Bartlett, 2005, p. 52.

52. Ibid.

53. Pfeiffer, R., and B. Mangus. *Concepts of Athletic Training*, 4th ed. Sudbury, MA: Jones and Bartlett, 2004, p. 265.

54. American Heart Association. http://www.americanheart.org/presenter.jhtml?identifier=2155.

55. American Council on Fitness. http://www.acefitness.org/fitfacts/fitfacts_display.aspx?itemid=57.

56. American Heart Association. http://www.americanheart.org.

57. *USA Today*, January 8, 2006. http://www.usatoday.com/news/health/2006-01-08-heart-nine-factors_x.htm.

58. American Heart Association. "Women and Heart Disease." http://www.americanheart.org/presenter.jhtml?identifier=2876.

59. American Heart Association. http://www.americanheart.org/presenter.jhtml?identifier=3053#Heart_Attack.

60. *New York Times*, January 9, 2006. http://www.nytimes.com/2006/01/09/nyregion/nyregionspecial5/09 diabetes.html?ei=5094&en=3a1180cac87d23c8&hp=&ex=1136869200&oref=login&partner=home page&pagewanted=print.

61. *New York Times*, January 9, 2006. http://www.nytimes.com/2006/01/09/nyregion/nyregionspecial5/09 diabetes.html?ei=5094&en=3a1180cac87d23c8&hp=&ex=1136869200&oref=login&partner=home page&pagewanted=print.

62. American Diabetes Association. http://www.diabetes.org/about-diabetes.jsp.

63. *New York Times*. "Guide to Knowledge." http://topics.nytimes.com/top/news/health/ diseasesconditionsandhealthtopics/bloodpressure/index.html?inline=nyt-classifier.

64. New York City Department of Health and Mental Hygiene. http://www.nyc.gov/health.

65. American Cancer Society. http://www.cancer.org.

66. National Cancer Institute. http://www.cancer.gov.

67. Ibid.

68. The Harvard Center for Cancer Prevention. http://www.yourdiseaserisk.harvard.edu/hccpquiz.pl?lang=english&func=show&quiz=breast&page=fact_sheet.

69. National Cancer Institute, U.S National Institutes of Health. http://www.Cancer.gov.

70. National Institutes of Health. http://www.nhlbi.nih.gov/health/dci/Diseases/Asthma/Asthma_WhatIs.html.

71. Ibid.

72. Food and Nutrition Board, Institute of Medicine, National Academies. *Dietary Reference Intakes: Application in Dietary Planning.* Washington, DC: National Academies Press, 2002.

73. University of Nebraska Cooperative Extension in Lancaster County. "Food Reflections," March 2004. http://lancaster.unl.edu/food/ftmar04.htm.

74. United States Department of Agriculture. "Food and Nutrition Information." http://www.nal.usda.gov/fnic/etext/ds_general.html.

75. *Dietary Guidelines for Americans,* 2005. http://www.healthierus.gov/dietaryguidelines/index.html.

76. Ibid.

77. Ibid.

78. National Heart, Lung, and Blood Institute. *Clinical Guidelines on the Identification, Evaluation, and Treatment of Obesity in Adults: The Evidence Report. NHLBI Obesity Education Initiative Expert Panel on the Identification, Evaluation, and Treatment of Obesity in Adults.* Washington, DC: U.S. Department of Health and Human Services, 1998.

79. American Obesity Association. *Shape Up America! Guidance for the Treatment of Adult Obesity.* Bethesda, MD: Author. Revised 1998.

80. Ibid.

81. National Institute of Diabetes and Digestive and Kidney Diseases. "Gastric Surgery for Severe Obesity." NIH Publication No. 96-4006, April 1996.

82. American Society for Bariatric Surgery. "Rationale for the Surgical Treatment of Obesity." April 6, 1998.

83. Renquist, K. "Obesity Classification." *Obesity Surgery,* Vol. 8, 1998, p. 480.

84. National Institutes of Health. "Consensus Development Conference Statement Online." *Gastrointestinal Surgery for Severe Obesity,* Vol. 1, March 25–27, 1999, pp. 1–20.

85. Kral, J. G. "Surgical Treatment of Obesity." In *Handbook of Obesity,* ed. G. A. Bray, C. Bouchard, and W. P. T. James. New York: Marcel Dekker, Inc., 1998.

86. FDA Talk Paper. "FDA Approves Implanted Stomach Band to Treat Severe Obesity." June 5, 2001.

87. American Society for Bariatric Surgery. "Rationale for the Surgical Treatment of Obesity." April 6, 1998.

88. American Psychiatric Association. *Diagnostic and Statistical Manual for Mental Disorders,* 4th ed. (APA): Washington DC: Author, 1994.

89. Ibid.

90. Hsu, G. L. K. "Epidemiology of the Eating Disorders." *Psychiatric Clinics of North America,* Vol. 19, No. 4, 1996, pp. 681–697.

91. Sullivan, P. F. "Mortality in Anorexia Nervosa." *American Journal of Psychiatry,* Vol. 152, 1995, pp. 1073–1074.

92. Zerbe, K. J. *The Body Betrayed.* Carlsbad, CA: Gurze Books, 1995.

93. American Psychiatric Association, *Diagnostic and Statistical Manual.*

94. Gidwani, G. P., and E. S. Rome. "Eating Disorders." *Clinical Obstetrics and Gynecology*, Vol. 40, No. 3, 1997, pp. 601–615.

95. Kendler, K. S., C. MacLean, M. Neale, R. Kessler, A. Heath, and L. Eaves. "The Genetic Epidemiology of Bulimia Nervosa." *American Journal of Psychiatry*, Vol. 148, 1991, pp. 1627–1637.

96. Zerbe, K. J. *The Body Betrayed.*

97. Smith, D. E., M. D. Marcus, C. E. Lewis, M. Fitzgibbon, and P. Schreiner. "Prevalence of Binge Eating Disorder, Obesity and Depression in a Biracial Cohort of Young Adults." *Annuls of Behavioral Medicine*, Vol. 20, pp. 227–232.

98. Ibid.

99. American Psychiatric Association, *Diagnostic and Statistical Manual.*

100. Ibid.

101. Ibid.

102. Henise, L., M. Ellsberg, and M. Geottemoeller. "Ending Violence Against Women." *Population Reports*, Series L, No. 11, December 1999.

103. National Center for Victim's Crime. http://www.ncvc.org.

104. Bureau of Justice Statistics. "Crime Data Brief, Intimate Partner Violence, 1993–2001." February, 2003.

105. Silverman, Jay G., Anita Raj, Lorelei A. Mucci, and Jeannie E. Hathaway. "Dating Violence Against Adolescent Girls and Associated Substance Use, Unhealthy Weight Control, Sexual Risk Behavior, Pregnancy, and Suicidality." *Journal of the American Medical Association*, Vol. 286, No. 5, 2001.

106. Bureau of Justice Statistics. "Violence Against Women: Estimates from the Redesigned Survey." August 1995.

107. Bureau of Justice Statistics. "Crime Data Brief, Intimate Partner Violence."

108. The National Domestic Violence Hotline. http://www.ndvh.org/educate/what_is_dv.html.

109. Ibid.

110. Ibid.

111. Ibid.

112. L. Walker. *The Battered Woman.* New York: Harper and Row, 1980.

113. Rennison, C. M. U.S. Department of Justice, Bureau of Justice Statistics. "Intimate Partner Violence and Age of the Victim, 1993–99." October 2001.

114. U.S. Department of Justice. "Prevalence, Incidence, and Consequences of Violence Against Women Survey," 1998.

115 Randall, M., and L. Haskell. "Sexual Violence in Women's Lives." *Violence Against Women*, Vol. 1, No. 1, 1995, pp. 6–31.

116. The National Women's Health Information Center. U.S Department of Health and Human Services. Office on Women's Health. http://womenshealth.gov/violence/sexual.cfm.

117. U.S. Department of Health and Human Services. National Institute on Alcohol Abuse and Alcoholism. *Journal: Alcohol Research & Health: Highlights from the Tenth Special Report to Congress, Health Risks and Benefits of Alcohol Consumption* (Volume 24, Number 1, 2000 ed.). Washington, DC: U.S. Government Printing Office. http://www.niaaa.nih.gov/publications/arh24-1/toc24-1.htm.

118. U.S. Department of Health and Human Services. Substance Abuse and Mental Health Services Administration. *Results from the 2001 National Household Survey on Drug Abuse: Volume I. Summary of National Findings* (Office of Applied Studies, NHSDA Series H-17 ed.) (BKD461, SMA 02-3758). Washington, DC: U.S. Government Printing Office, 2002. http://www.oas.samhsa.gov/nhsda/2k1nhsda/vol1/Chapter3.htm.

119. U.S. Department of Health and Human Services. SAMHSA's Center for Substance Abuse Treatment. *You Can Help: A Guide for Caring Adults Working with Young People Experiencing Addiction in the Family* (PHD878, (SMA) 01-3544). Washington, DC: U.S. Government Printing Office. http://www.samhsa.gov/centers/csat/content/intermediaries.

120. Ibid.

121. AMA. http://www.ama-assn.org/ama/pub/category/13246.html.

122. Center on Alcohol Marketing and Youth, January 2006. http://camy.org/factsheets/index.php?FactsheetID=7.

123. Hingson, R., et al. "Magnitude of Alcohol-Related Mortality and Morbidity Among U.S. College Students Ages 18–24: Changes from 1998 to 2001." *Annual Review of Public Health*, Vol. 26, 2005, pp. 259–279.

124. Snyder, L. B., F. F. Milici, M. Slater, H. Sun, and Y. Strizhakova. "Effects of Alcohol Advertising Exposure on Drinking Among Youth." *Archives of Pediatrics and Adolescent Medicine*, Vol. 160, 2006, pp. 18–24.

125. Strasburger, V. C., and E. Donnerstein. "Children, Adolescents, and the Media: Issues and Solutions." *Pediatrics*, Vol. 103, No. 1, 1999, pp. 129–139.

126. Adams Business Media. *Beer Handbook*. Norwalk, CT: Author, 2001.

127. Chura, H., and W. Friedman. "Diageo Moves Forward with Network Plan: Marketer to Run $200 Million in Liquor Ads on TV Consortium." *Advertising Age*, May 13, 2000.

128. Jernigan, D., and P. Wright, eds. *Making News, Changing Policy: Using Media Advocacy to Change Alcohol and Tobacco Policy*. Rockville, MD: Center for Substance Abuse Prevention, 1994; B. Gallegos, *Chasing the Frogs and Camels out of Los Angeles: The Movement to Limit Alcohol and Tobacco Billboards: A Case Study*. San Rafael, CA: The Marin Institute for the Prevention of Alcohol and Other Drug Problems, 1999.

129. J. M. Wallace Jr., et al. "The Epidemiology of Alcohol, Tobacco and Other Drug Use Among Black Youth." *Journal of Studies on Alcohol*, Vol. 60, 1999, pp. 800–809.

130. Substance Abuse and Mental Health Services Administration. *Results from the 2004 National Survey on Drug Use and Health: National Findings*. Rockville, MD: Office of Applied Studies, 2005, table H.25.

131. Centers for Disease Control and Prevention (CDC). "Annual Smoking-Attributable Mortality, Years of Potential Life Lost, and Economic Costs—United States, 1995–1999." *MMWR*. Vol. 51, 2002, pp. 300–303. http://www.cdc.gov/mmwr//preview/mmwrhtml/mm5114a2.htm.

132. American Cancer Society. *Cancer Facts & Figures 2005*. Atlanta, GA: American Cancer Society, 2005.

133. http://www.drugabuse.gov/Infofax/tobacco.html.

134. American Cancer Society, *Cancer Facts & Figures 2005*.

135. Ibid.

136. Ibid.

137. Office of the U.S. Surgeon General. "The Health Consequences of Smoking: Nicotine Addiction: A Report of the Surgeon General, Centers for Disease Control and Prevention (CDC), Office on Smoking and Health. 1988." http://www.cdc.gov/tobacco/sgr/sgr_1988/index.htm.

138. Office of the U.S. Surgeon General. "The Health Benefits of Smoking Cessation: A Report of the Surgeon General, Centers for Disease Control and Prevention (CDC), Office on Smoking and Health. 1990." http://profiles.nlm.nih.gov/NN/B/B/C/T/.

139. U.S. Department of Health and Human Services. Substance Abuse and Mental Health Services Administration. *Understanding Drug Abuse and Addiction: What Science Says: Slide Teaching Packet III, for Health Practitioners, Teachers and Neuroscientists* (AVD145). Washington, DC: U.S. Government Printing Office, 2001. http://www.drugabuse.gov/Teaching3/Teaching.html.

140. U.S. Department of Health and Human Services. Substance Abuse and Mental Health Services Administration. *Summary of Findings from the 2000 National Household Survey on Drug Abuse* (Office of Applied Studies, NHSDA Series H-13 ed.) ([SMA] 01-3549). Washington, DC: U.S. Government Printing Office, 2002. http://www.samhsa.gov/oas/nhsda/2knhsda/chapter2.

141. http://www.drugabuse.gov/Infofax/marijuana.html.

142. U.S. Department of Health and Human Services. SAMHSA's Center for Substance Abuse Prevention. *Prevention Alert: Club Drugs: A New Community Threat* (Volume 3, Number 24 ed.). Washington, DC: U.S. Government Printing Office. http://ncadi.samhsa.gov/govpubs/prevalert/v3i24.aspx.

143. U.S. Department of Health and Human Services. National Institute on Drug Abuse. *NIDA InfoFacts: MDMA (Ecstasy)*. Washington, DC: U.S. Government Printing Office, 2002. http://www.drugabuse.gov/Infofax/ecstasy.html.

144. U.S. Department of Health and Human Services. National Institute on Drug Abuse. *NIDA Info Facts: Rohypnol and GHB*. Washington, DC: U.S. Government Printing Office, 2002. http://www.nida.nih.gov/Infofax/RohypnolGHB.html.

145. U.S. Department of Health and Human Services. SAMHSA's Center for Substance Abuse Prevention. *Prevention Alert: Club Drugs: GHB, an Anabolic Steroid* (Volume 3, Number 27 ed.). Washington, DC: U.S. Government Printing Office. http://ncadi.samhsa.gov/govpubs/prevalert/v3i27.aspx.

146. U.S. Department of Health and Human Services. National Institute on Drug Abuse. *NIDA Research Report: Methamphetamine Abuse and Addiction*. Washington, DC: U.S. Government Printing Office, 2002. http://www.drugabuse.gov/ResearchReports/methamph/methamph2.html#what.

147. http://www.drugabuse.gov/Infofax/methamphetamine.html.

148. Breggin, P. *Talking Back to Ritalin: What Doctors Aren't Telling You About Stimulants for Children*. Monroe, ME: Common Courage Press, 1998.

149. Breggin, P. *Reclaiming Our Children: A Healing Solution for a Nation in Crisis*. Cambridge, MA: Perseus Books, 2000.

150. U.S. Department of Health and Human Services. National Institute on Drug Abuse. *NIDA InfoFacts: Heroin*. Washington, DC: U.S. Government Printing Office, 2002. http://www.drugabuse.gov/Infofax/heroin.html.

151. http://www.drugabuse.gov/Infofax/heroin.html.

152. U.S. Department of Health and Human Services. National Institute on Drug Abuse. *NIDA Research Report—Cocaine Abuse and Addiction* (PHD813, NIH Publication No. 99-4342). Washington, DC: U.S. Government Printing Office, 2002. http://www.drugabuse.gov/ResearchReports/Cocaine/cocaine2.html#what.

153. http://www.drugabuse.gov/Infofax/cocaine.html.

154. U.S. Department of Health and Human Services. National Institute on Drug Abuse. *NIDA InfoFacts: Inhalants*. Washington, DC: U.S. Government Printing Office, 2002. http://www.drugabuse.gov/Infofax/inhalants.html.

155. Centers for Disease Control and Prevention. http://www.cdc.gov/std.

156. Centers for Disease Control and Prevention. "Sexually Transmitted Diseases Treatment Guidelines 2002." *MMWR* Vol. 51, 2002 (no. RR-6).

157. Koutsky, L. A., and N. B. Kiviat. Genital human papillomavirus. In *Sexually Transmitted Diseases*, 3rd ed., K. Holmes, P. Sparling, P. Mardh et al. (eds). New York: McGraw-Hill, 1999, pp. 347–359.

158. American Social Health Association. http://www.ashastd.org.

159. Ibid.

160. Centers for Disease Control and Prevention. *Sexually Transmitted Disease Surveillance, 2002*. Atlanta, GA: U.S. Department of Health and Human Services, September 2003.

161. Holmes, K., P. Mardh, P. Sparling, et al. (eds). *Sexually Transmitted Diseases*, 3rd ed. New York: McGraw-Hill, 1999, chapters 33–37.

162. Centers for Disease Control and Prevention. "Sexually Transmitted Diseases Treatment Guidelines 2002." *MMWR* Vol. 51, 2002. (no. RR-6).

163. Ibid.

164. National Herpes Resource Center and Hotline. American Social Health Association. http://www.ashastd.org/hrc/index.html.

165. Epigee Women's Health. http://www.epigee.org.

166. *New York Times*, Tuesday, January 31, 2006.

167. National Campaign to Prevent Teen Pregnancy analysis of Henshaw, S. K., *U.S. Teenage Pregnancy Statistics*. New York: Alan Guttmacher Institute, 1996.

168. Singh, S., and J. E. Darroch. "Adolescent Pregnancy and Childbearing: Levels and Trends in Developed Countries." *Family Planning Perspectives*, Vol. 32, No. 1, 2000, pp. 14–23.

169. Infectious Diseases Society of America. http://www.idsa.org.

170. National Institute of Allergy and Infectious Diseases. http://www.niaid.nih.gov/publications/microbes.htm#a.

171. Ibid.

172. Ibid.

173. Centers for Disease Control and Prevention, National Center for HIV, STD, and TB Prevention. http://www.cdc.gov/hiv/pubs/faq/faq17.htm.

174. Glynn, M., and P. Rhodes. "Estimated HIV Prevalence in the United States at the End of 2003." National HIV Prevention Conference, June 2005, Atlanta, GA. Abstract 595.

175. *New York Times*, February 4, 2006.

176. AIDS info. http://aidsinfo.nih.gov/.

CPSIA information can be obtained
at www.ICGtesting.com
Printed in the USA
LVHW020855200619
621712LV00003B/5/P